DEPARTMENT OF HEALTH AND SOCIAL SECURITY
OFFICE OF THE CHIEF SCIENTIST

RESEARCH REPORT NO 12

Costs and Benefits of the Heart Transplant Programmes at Harefield and Papworth Hospitals

Martin Buxton
Roy Acheson
Noreen Caine
Stuart Gibson
Bernie O'Brien

LONDON: HER MAJESTY'S STATIONERY OFFICE

ISBN 0 11 321033 7

The views expressed in this report are not necessarily those of the
Department of Health and Social Security

Preface

This *Report* to the Department of Health and Social Security summarises the findings of a three year study by our Research Team, from the Department of Economics at Brunel University and the Department of Community Medicine at Cambridge. It follows two earlier Reports to the DHSS — a *Preliminary Report* at the end of 1982 and an *Interim Report* in the autumn of 1983. It was not appropriate to publish these, and therefore this document has been written as a free-standing account of the work. For reasons of length we cannot spell out in detail here all the developmental work and exploratory analysis we have carried out. Where we believe this to be of interest to other researchers we aim to publishers more detailed papers in appropriate scientific journals.

Even so we are aware that for some of the widely differing readers likely to be interested in this *Report* particular Chapters may seem rather technical. We have therefore endeavoured to present non-technical summaries at the end of each Chapter and, together with the final Chapter as a whole, these provide a brief summary of the *Report*. It is important to stress however that these summaries inevitably omit the many caveats and cautions that are indicated in the main body of the Chapters. Such caveats, nevertheless, should not be ignored and the rather bald statements in the summaries must be treated cautiously.

It is also important to stress that the Report and its findings should be ascribed solely to the Research Team, and should not be taken as necessarily the views of any of the other parties involved in the programmes, or who have assisted us in any way.

The Research Team has been given an immense amount of co-operation. Indeed the success of a two-centre study of this scale and breadth relies on the help and goodwill of a great number of people. The involvement of Mr Magdi Yaccoub and Mr Terence English, and his colleagues Mr Richard Cory-Pearce and Mr John Wallwork, has been essential at all stages in the study; their help has been generously given, and mere acknowledgement seems totally inadequate. But they, like others, may wish to disagree with the implications of our findings.

At various stages, particularly in determining the methodology we sought advice from many experts who readily gave of their time, experience and wisdom. We would like in particular to thank: Mr Douglas Harper, Dr Alex Barr, Mrs Pauline Rogers, Dr Brian Moores, Mr Leonard Goldstone, Ms Margaret Collier, and Dr Barbara Wade for their advice on measuring nursing time and patient dependency; Dr Rita Redberg for her earlier work on measuring medical time; Dr Rory Williams, Dr Donald Patrick, Dr Jim McEwen, and Dr Sonja Hunt, for advice on measuring health status; Professor David Cox and Dr David Oakes, Dr Carolyn Dore, Professor Peter Armitage and Dr Vern Farewell for their advice on the survival analysis; Professor John Goodwin and Professor Geoffrey Rose for comments on the epidemiology; and Dr Roger Evans for providing information from the National Heart Transplantation Study in the U.S.A.

Many of our colleagues at Brunel and Cambridge Universities have given witting or unwitting advice and have been used as sounding-boards for our ideas. The Research Team also wish to thank Ms Alex Morris, who was very actively involved in the earlier stages of the project at Papworth, and who carried out amongst other valuable work, some of the studies of medical time. We also owe sincere thanks to our various clerical and secretarial support — particularly Mrs Shirley Buckland, Miss Alison Munt, Miss Susan Evans, and Mrs Jo Patterson. A paticualr debt is due to Mrs Mary Elliott who has typed the many drafts of this and the earlier reports and has had to cope with our impossible time-tables and demands.

Finally there are two large groups from whom it would be invidious to pick out specific individuals. We should like to thank *all* those members of the staff of the two hospitals, and their District Authorities, who directly or indirectly have helped in offering assistance, providing data, or merely cheerfully tolerating our presence. Last, but certainly not least, the patients involved — who have answered our repeated questionnaires, filled in diaries, and co-operated in the interviews — must receive our thanks. We hope they recognise the picture they have helped us to paint.

MARTIN BUXTON
February 1985

Contents

1. Introduction and Background to the Study

1.1 Terms of reference and organisation of the study

At the end of October 1981, DHSS research funds were granted to the Department of Economics, Brunel University, and the Department of Community Medicine, University of Cambridge, to carry out co-ordinated studies of the costs and benefits of the cardiac transplant programmes at Harefield and Papworth Hospitals over a three year period. The research was intended to "identify, and carry out a detailed analysis of, the resource requirements and thus the costs of the current heart transplant programmes at Papworth and Harefield Hospitals and to relate these to appropriate indicators of patient benefits". The study was seen as having three main elements:

(1) The analysis of resource costs within Papworth and Harefield Hospitals associated with their respective transplant programmes;

(2) the identification and analysis of extra NHS costs and other public sector costs incurred outside the two centres by patients involved in the transplant programmes and their selection procedures;

(3) the measurement of benefits in terms of basic outcome data.

The results were to be analysed and presented, "to show the position with respect to both centres individually and in terms of a more generalised statement drawing on data from both."

It was decided not to attempt a formal study of the epidemiology of present and future demand for heart transplantation, although a brief consideration of the topic is included in this *Report* as contextual background to the main evaluation.

A considerable amount of preliminary work on research instruments and methods had already been undertaken by the Cambridge team on the Papworth programme. This work had been supported by the East Anglian Regional Health Authority during the period October 1980 – October 1981.

Although the DHSS research protocol provided for three reports, to be presented at yearly intervals, it was agreed that only this, the *Final Report*, would be published.

The original research protocol clearly recognised the uncertainty about the continued funding of the two transplant programmes. At that time their funding was only assured until the end of December 1982 (at Papworth) and the end of March 1983 (at Harefield).

The research protocol therefore provided for two alternative patterns of study:

(a) in the event of the non-extension of the programmes, *faut de mieux* a considerable reliance would have to be put on retrospective collection and analysis of data pertaining to the earlier parts of the programmes prior to the setting-up of the research; or

(b) the preferred option, possible only if the programmes were extended, was

1

for the analysis to be based almost exclusively on prospectively collected data.

In the event, financial support from the DHSS has been given to each of the surgical programmes on an ad-hoc basis. This funding has permitted their continuation, albeit on a rather insecure basis, and has enabled the research team to implement its preferred plan to rely on prospective data collection. Thus with the exception of some general data on the magnitude of the programmes (presented in Chapter 2) and basic survival data for the early part of the programmes (used in Chapter 8) no retrospective data has been used.

The formal protocol established two parallel but co-ordinated studies of the programmes at Harefield and Papworth. In practice the level of co-ordination and integration of our research has been such that it has effectively been a single study of the two centres' transplant programmes. However it is important to stress that these two programmes are quite independent and, whilst in many ways they are very similar, there are some detailed but nevertheless important differences between them in clinical management, in available resources and in institutional background. We have tried to indicate these, where we believe them to be of relevance to our study.

1.2 The methodological framework of the study

In reading, interpreting, and evaluating this Report, the context in which the study was set up should be borne in mind. Both programmes were already in existence and had been established quite independently. They straddled the boundary between what might be termed clinical research and a routine (albeit highly specialised) patient service. The programmes do not constitute a formal clinical trial, a fact which has raised difficult problems in evaluating them.

In a preliminary report on the background to the concurrent National Heart Transplantation Study in the United States, it is suggested that the following question has to be addressed: — "What costs associated with medical and surgical management of an end-stage cardiac disease patient would have been incurred regardless of whether a heart transplant was performed?" It goes on, "The emphasis should be on the economic and social costs of end-stage cardiac disease treated by two methods: (1) conventional medical and surgical therapy, and (2) heart transplantation." (Evans [1982a])

Our study similarly aims to try to identify the extra costs and benefits resulting from the existence of the cardiac transplant programmes as compared to those of conventional medical and surgical therapy. This is the appropriate comparison on which to judge whether or not the extra costs are justified, and hence the comparison that should influence the policy decision concerning the future of cardiac transplantation.

The agreed protocol for the study recognised that we would not be able to quantify, nor indeed consider in great detail, all relevant cost and benefit differences. Two omissions need to be stressed. Firstly, we have not specifically measured the private costs to the individual patient, his family or employer. Nor have we attempted to assess the non-direct patient benefits of the programmes in terms of the research value of these "experimental" programmes to the care of future cardiac patients, nor the spin-off value to other groups of patients, nor indeed the value of greater understanding and scientific knowledge *per se*.

However in other ways we are taking a broad view of the costs. We take the programme as encompassing all the stages from referral to the transplant centre to the continuing follow-up of patients transplanted. Much of the early discussion of the resource requirements and costs of heart transplantation has focussed too narrowly on the recipient operation and the immediate postoperative care. In particular, early work has failed to take full account of the costs of assessment for *all* patients assessed regardless of outcome and any other extra costs incurred by accepted patients who die whilst waiting for a transplant operation. (See for example: Haberman [1980]; Hellinger [1982].) Even Evans [1982a], in a generally very thorough study of the costs of heart transplantation, appears to consider only the costs for those who receive a transplant.

Equally important is the necessity of clearly defining the *extra* elements of patient care and treatment (and hence extra resource-usage and costs) that result from the existence of the programme. Some of the potential confusion surrounding this issue stems from the fact that this study has no formal set of controls consisting of traditionally managed patients for comparison. Unfortunately, from the point of view of our evaluation the programmes were not set up in an orthodox experimental manner with a randomised control group. Indeed in the strict sense not even an acceptable non-randomised control group exists against which to compare the costs and benefits of the transplanted patients.

In the absence of proper controls the study had to obtain as much relevant comparative information as possible from the various patient groups accessible to the researchers. FIGURE 1.1 represents a decision tree indicating the basic possible outcomes for any patients within the total population suffering from relevant heart disease. If thus defines the major patient sub-groups relevant to this study. (The letters of the branches of this diagram are used as reference points to the particular patient groups in the text below.)

Of the total population with heart disease of the types that might possibly be treated by transplantation (U), some will be referred to either centre (A). The others who are not referred (B) remain unidentified and unknown to the researchers. (Using routine national data Chapter Eleven explores the possible size of the population who might potentially be relevantly referred for heart transplantation.) Some referrals are considered unsuitable on the basis of the clinical criteria discussed in the next Chapter and therefore not called for assessment (D). In practical terms, though identifiable, they are not a group that is easily accessible to the researchers.

Therefore in practice the population that we could "monitor" in this study was the assessment population (C), and we attempted to collect information on all patients in this group. Once a decision is made after assessment, this group splits into two — (E) accepted for transplant (both "definitely" and "provisionally") and (F) not accepted for transplant. At any point in time those accepted (who are still alive) are either transplanted (G) or waiting (H). A few of those not accepted, as a result of the assessment, are given an alternative operation (I). The others return to their previous medical regime (J).

1.3 Benefit comparisons

In considering the *benefits* of transplantation, *ideally* we required a control group of patients who were clinically strictly comparable to those accepted for transplant, but who were randomly allocated to continuing medical therapy. In

Figure 1.1: Basic decision tree diagram for a cardiac transplantation programme

Key

☐ Decision points

■ Decision points including added uncertainty of donor heart availability

U,A...J Population descriptors

PA ... PJ Transition probabilities for each population sub group (eg. PA + PB = 1)

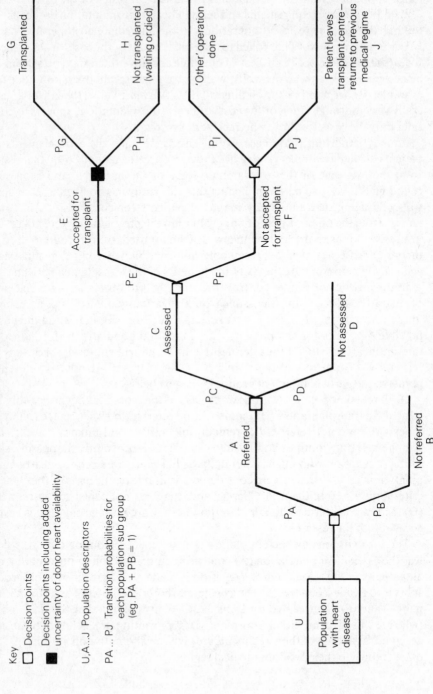

4

the absence of orthodox controls, a sub-group within (J) such as those rejected on purely psychosocial grounds or because they were just outside the age limits, might have provided suitable comparisons; in practice any such sub-group was too small to be useful. Group (J) as a *whole* however will include patients who are very different from the transplanted patients in (G). Moreover they were for obvious reasons the group of assessed patients with the weakest clinical links with the transplant centres, and a very difficult group to monitor for this study.

Thus the main group against which comparisons can be made is group (H). Even this is not without problems in that the patients who die from that group *may* tend to be the iller patients for whom a suitable donor heart is not available in time. The patients still waiting at any point in time *may* tend to be those with the relatively better prognosis who have not been put at the top of the "waiting list".

In short, any comparisons between sub-groups must be made with extreme caution and all reasons for differences between them explored. Chapter Eight describes, for example, some of the problems that relate to the appropriate use of survival data from (H) as a control for (G). Similarly Chapter Nine utilises the same comparisons of subjective health status information. Such comparisons are essential to the estimation of the "extra" benefits from transplantation as compared with existing "routine" management.

1.4 Cost comparisons

In terms of the analysis of costs it is even more difficult to identify correctly the *extra* costs. For example, it would clearly be inappropriate to include in the costs of a transplant programme *all* costs of care for those waiting for transplant, because in the absence of a programme they would still be receiving medical care. We need to identify what extra costs are incurred *because* the patient is awaiting transplant.

The obvious approach would have been to measure the total cost of a patient period in group (H) and deduct the total costs of an equivalent patient period in group (J). However, even if one accepts the validity of the cost comparison between the two groups, the small numbers of patients involved combined with the complexity of costing patients in a variety of different situations, at home or in hospital anywhere in the UK, puts grave doubts on the significance of any cost difference so measured. The cost differences observed might equally well be the product of cost estimating or cost sampling problems, or simply random differences reflecting the particular patients or hospitals concerned.

A more practicable alternative is to identify specifically any costs that are additional (viz extra costs resulting from the existence of the transplant programmes). For example, during the "waiting period" (between acceptance onto the programme after assessment and transplantation/death), we have attempted to distinguish those costs that would not have been incurred had the patient not been referred and accepted. Obviously the costs of any "monitoring" by the transplant teams keeping in touch with patients and their referring doctors can fairly easily be identified and accounted for. But in addition, we need to identify what other differences, *if any*, in treatment (such as drug regimes, routine tests, consultant attendances, lengths of in-patient stay) potential transplant patients typically receive. These extra costs are considered further in Chapter Seven.

1.5 The importance of the cost and benefit data

It has often been suggested to us that what we should be focussing on directly is the impact of the transplant programmes on the hospitals, particularly any effect on their "normal" or "pre-existing" workloads. Examples have been cited to us both of the pressures created on some staff, particularly as a result of the unpredictable but mainly out-of-hours timing of the transplant operations, and the effect on "routine" theatre lists by the unplanned daytime use of theatres or use by transplant patients of ITU beds.

It has never been our aim or remit to measure the consequences of introducing a transplant programme in terms of staff or patient morale or the detailed organisational impact on the hospitals. A quite different mode of research and a different team of researchers would have been required, and at the end of the exercise the results, though fascinating, would be highly particular to the circumstances of Harefield and Papworth during the period of the study, to the specific personalities, attitudes and relationships of their staffs, but of little use in helping to determine future priorities for expenditure within the NHS.

We have focussed on the costs and benefits in that the costs provide a convenient short-hand for the forgone alternative uses of the resources. They provide a measuring rod for the variety of alternative ways in which the resources might have been used. In the short term, and in a local perspective, the costs measure the resources that could, financial arrangements permitting, be used for alternative "routine" cardiac surgery. In the longer term, and from a national perspective, they can be taken as an indication of the value of resources that would be absorbed by the programmes that might otherwise be used for a quite different service within the NHS. This process of comparing benefits achieved with benefits foregone via the costs would of course be a lot easier if more studies were available using data comparable to those collected here. (We return to this issue of comparative costs and benefits in Chapter Twelve.)

1.6 The structure of the *Report*

Our *Report* attempts within limits of reasonable length to present a full account of the main aspects of our research. All material relating to the heart-lung transplant elements of the programmes has been excluded from the analysis. The *Report* is structured in four sections:

SECTION I provides a background to the size and nature of the two programmes, presents data on the characteristics of the patients involved and summarises information on the overall use of resources in the two hospitals.

SECTION II deals with the costs by presenting the arguments for our costing concepts, the details of the costing conventions that underlay our unit costs, and by summarising the data on the costs of patients within the programmes.

SECTION III presents the information on benefits to patients in terms of survival and quality of life — the latter being expressed in terms of both statistical data obtained by using a standardised questionnaire on patients' subjective health states and the more impressionistic but vivid account based on interviews.

Finally, SECTION IV draws these elements together, puts them into the overall context of the epidemiological picture and presents them in such a way that the costs and benefits of heart transplantation can begin to be related to alternative uses of the resources. This section attempts somewhat speculatively to consider the future of such programmes and to draw out some of the implications.

1.7 Summary

Funds for this three year study were made available in the Autumn of 1981 to the Department of Economics, Brunel University, and the Department of Community Medicine, University of Cambridge. The closely co-ordinated studies of the two programmes have effectively amounted to a single evaluation, although the surgical programmes themselves are quite independent.

The three main elements of the research were the analysis of the resource costs associated with the transplant programmes at Harefield and Papworth hospitals; the identification of the extra NHS costs and other public sector costs incurred outside the two centres, and the measurement of the direct benefits derived by patients in terms of survival and quality of life. We have costed the programme defined broadly, from initial patient referral to the transplant centres to the long-term care of patients who have received transplants. We have looked at the benefits in terms of a service to current patients and not in terms of any research value. The study has focussed on the costs of resources as a measure of the opportunities forgone elsewhere, as distinct from trying to identify any specific impact on the other patients or other activities of the hospitals, or on staff morale.

The bulk of the data has been collected prospectively, and to present as comprehensive a picture as possible within the three year study, we have looked not only at cohorts of new patients but also at the quality of life and costs of care during the period of our study of patients transplanted prior to its commencement.

The most fundamental limitation of the study from the point of view of the conduct of the research, and the analysis and interpretation of our results, was that because it was unacceptable to randomly allocate patients between surgery and a conventional medical regime, no formal control group existed. In its absence our comparisons are principally, but not exclusively, with patients who though accepted for transplantation had not received a transplant. These comparisons, although illuminating, must be interpreted cautiously.

2. The Nature of the Programmes and Basic Programme Data

2.1 Introduction

As has already been noted, the two programmes are fundamentally similar and it is quite reasonable to present a common statement of their main stages and characteristics. Against this background we set the data on the size of the programmes, the main characteristics of the referral, assessment and transplant recipient populations, and of the sources of donor hearts.

2.2 The general nature of the programmes

The following account, together with the diagramatic presentation in FIGURE 2.1 provide a brief generalised statement of the main stages in the transplant programme as seen from the point of view of an individual's possible progress through it.

Referral

The selection of patients for cardiac transplant is effectively a two stage screening procedure of referral and assessment. Typically the patient will initially have consulted both his local GP and a hospital consultant who may then exercise the option of referral to either of the transplant centres for consideration for heart transplant. The majority of referrals have been made by cardiologists and physicians, and some by other cardiac surgeons. A few have come direct from GPs, from patients' relatives, or from patients themselves.

On most occasions the referral process is clear and specific. A written request, or an initial telephone request confirmed in writing, is made usually by a doctor in a hospital elsewhere. However, in a few instances the situation may be less clear cut, for example:

(a) A few patients seen by Mr Yacoub are new local patients or long-standing Harefield cardiac patients for whom he may now introduce the possibility of transplantation being an appropriate treatment.

(b) A few patients have been referred to Mr Yacoub for his views as to the possibility of further surgery without explicit reference or implicit focus on transplantation. For these again, transplantation will inevitably be one of a range of possible surgical procedures that he will implicitly or explicitly consider.

(c) Certain emergency admissions from other centres have been considered for transplantation without a formal process of referral.

Assessment

At this referral stage the patient has usually undergone a series of routine tests and often more specific cardiological tests at his local hospital. On the basis of a summary of this information usually contained in the referral letter, the trans-

8

Figure 2.1: A simplified flow chart of the stages involved in a heart transplant programme

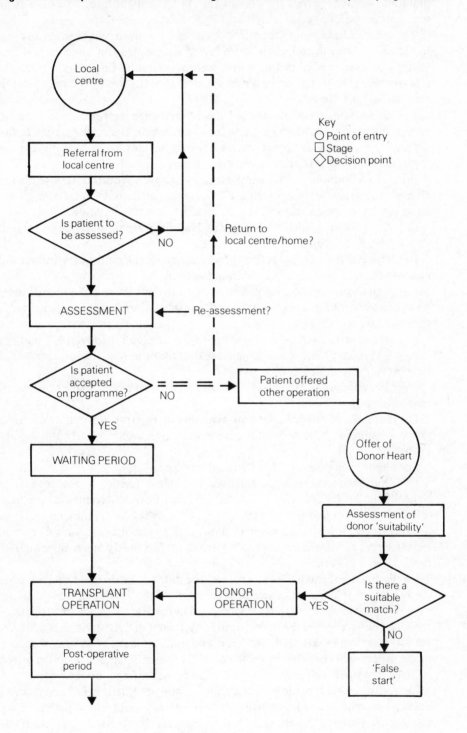

9

plant surgeons decide whether or not the patient is possibly suitable for transplant and whether or not the patient should be brought into the centre as an inpatient for definitive assessment.

The decision to bring in the patient for assessment or to reject him as unsuitable at this stage will reflect the criteria for acceptance for transplant. These criteria, as then applied at Papworth, were spelt out by English, Cooper, and Cory-Pearce [1980]. The criteria now applicable to the two programmes can be summarised as follows:

(i) All potential recipients should have "end stage" cardiac disease due to irreversible myocardial damage secondary to Ischaemic Heart Disease or Cardiomyopathy (occasionally other causes), which cannot be treated by further medical therapy or conventional cardiac surgery.

(ii) Raised Pulmonary Vascular Resistance (above 8 Wood Units) is seen as an absolute contraindication of suitability for an orthotopic heart transplant, although a heterotopic transplant is an alternative in this situation.

(iii) The general guidelines for age at Harefield are up to 59 years, and at Papworth 15 – 50 years.

(iv) There should be no active infection nor recent pulmonary infarction; however these are not absolute contraindications.

(v) With the advent of Cyclosporin A, insulin dependent diabetes mellitus is no longer a contraindication, but the patients should be free of the other complications of diabetes.

(vi) Impairment of renal and hepatic function should be reversible and not caused by primary disease affecting these organs, otherwise a transplant would be contraindicated.

(vii) They should be psychosocially stable and with a reasonable prospect of rehabilitation.

On the basis of the information available at referral, an initial screening process excludes those for whom transplantation would clearly not be appropriate.

Four important points of detail should be noted:

(a) Whilst the tests required and used to make a decision at assessment are basically similar for the two centres, there are significant differences in the extent to which they require (and use) tests carried out by the local referring centre in advance of admission for assessment. Papworth has a policy of requiring certain tests to be carried out in advance. Mr Yacoub prefers to rely much more on tests carried out at Harefield.

(b) Following the assessment process, the date of the decision to accept the patient or not is a crucial benchmark for some of the survival analyses. In the case of some of the early assessments carried out at Harefield, where the patient remained as a patient in the hospital, the exact point of acceptance is not always entirely clear from the records available, and some estimating has been necessary in retrospectively considering these cases. Only rarely has the problem arisen with the "prospective" patients observed since the study got underway.

(c) A distinction is made between patients who are "definitely" and "provisionally" accepted. For Papworth, where a greater proportion of patients have been "provisionally" accepted, a clear dividing line has been specified thus: "If at the time of assessment the immediate prognosis is not considered bad enough to warrant transplantation, the patient may be placed in a "provisional" category, whereby he is closely followed up by the referring cardiologist and only accepted definitely if further deterioration takes place.'' (English [1982]) At Harefield the ''provisional'' designation is rarely used.

(d) Some patients referred to Papworth have been assessed by one of the transplant surgeons in the referring hospital because the patients were too ill to be transferred. The small number of assessments carried out outside Harefield have taken place mainly at the National Heart Hospital to which Mr Yacoub is jointly appointed.

Those considered suitable for formal assessment are normally brought into the centre for an inpatient stay to undergo a predetermined set of tests and assessments, on the basis of which a decision is made whether to offer to accept the patient onto the programme or to reject the patient, or, relatively rarely, to offer the patient alternative cardiac surgery.

Waiting Period

Those selected for transplant then face a period of waiting. Depending on the patient's immediate state of health, his home location, etc, he may either wait at home, in his local hospital or at the transplant centre until such time as a suitable donor-heart becomes available for him. Throughout this period, patients are monitored for any change in condition that may alter their suitability for transplant.

During the ''waiting period'', patients at the two centres have experienced rather different arrangements. In almost all cases after assessment Papworth has discharged the patient to his home if well enough, or to his local/referring centre. At Harefield it has been much more common for the patient to ''wait'' at Harefield, if too ill to be returned home; the proportion waiting at Harefield has however declined considerably.

Donors

The criteria for selection, and the process of procurement of hearts for transplantation, have been set out in English *et al* [1984]. The current criteria can be summarised as follows:

(i) Hearts from patients older than 35 years are not usually accepted because of the prevalence of undetected coronary disease in the general population.

(ii) Compatability of the size of the heart between recipient and donor is occasionally a consideration for orthotopic transplantation, but donors aged less than 15 can be used for heterotopic transplantation as well as for orthotopic transplantation in other adults who do not have significant pulmonary hypertension.

(iii) ABO blood group compatability is essential.

(iv) Cross matching of donor lymphocytes and recipient serum is not necessary, except in those patients who are known to have cytotoxic antibodies, following tests at assessment.

(v) Tissue typing is performed on all recipients and donors, but at present HLA including DR mismatching is not regarded as a contraindication.

(vi) Relevant medical information about the donor is obtained by telephone at the time of referral. There should be no history of cardiac disease, systemic infection, malignancy other than primary cerebral tumour, or of being on long-term medication.

11

All donors have suffered irreversible brain damage, usually as a result of road traffic accidents or intracranial haemorrhage. The diagnosis of brain death is made by doctors who are independent of the transplant team. In some cases the transplant centre is informed of a possible donor heart by a surgical team who have obtained permission to remove the donor's kidneys for transplantation or by UK Transplant acting on similar information. The UK Transplant Service is a co-ordinating body whose primary function is "the acquisition and redistribution of transplantable organs". Listings of potential recipients are kept by their office in Bristol, and they also endeavour to provide communication, information and laboratory services. (UK Transplant Service [1982])

The teams at the transplant centres then determine which patient from their waiting list should receive the donor heart. Within the constraints of the criteria set out above, the heart is normally allocated to whichever patient has been waiting longest. However occasionally a donor heart may be used for a recipient who has been on the waiting list for a shorter length of time if it is known that he or she is deteriorating rapidly.

The chosen recipient is immediately brought into the transplant centre for preparation. The donor operation is timed to start in accordance with the necessary preparation of the recipient after admission to the centre. A team from the transplant centre proceeds to the donor hospital to remove the heart. Close contact is maintained throughout and when the donor heart is safely excised, the word is given by telephone to begin the recipient operation.

Transplant Operation

The donor heart is brought back to the centre as quickly as possible, usually by a combination of road and air transport. It is taken straight into theatre where the recipient will already have been prepared for the operation. Prior to this the patient will have begun to receive the various immunosuppressive drugs to diminish the possibility of rejection of the donor heart.

Postoperative Care

Postoperatively the patient is transferred to a single room attached to ITU and reverse barrier nursing is carried out. This regime is maintained for the first few days to reduce the risks of infection whilst immunosuppression is at its maximum. Subsequently the patient can be managed with normal ward care.

During this period rehabilitation is continued with daily physiotherapy sessions and the patient is taught how to take his own drugs and is instructed on diet.

After discharge the patient is seen on a regular and frequent basis as an outpatient both at the transplant centre and the patient's referring centre. Biopsies of the heart are carried out at regular intervals to detect any signs of rejection. At the anniversary of the operation a full cardiological investigation is carried out. Any problems of infection or indications of rejection are likely to lead to readmission as an inpatient.

The Harefield programme has the use of three flats in Harefield village which are paid for by the Harefield Heart Transplant Trust, and used by patients who do not live locally, for a period immediately after discharge when daily outpatient visits are required for routine monitoring. Arrangements are now made for

Papworth patients to be found accommodation locally when they return for tests, to avoid the necessity of admission as inpatients. Occasionally, for patients whose home is particularly far from Papworth, similar accommodation has been found for a week or two immediately following discharge.

2.3 Basic programme data (as at 30 September 1984)

In that our own prospective data collection began early in 1982, data for the period prior to this (1979–81) had to be collected retrospectively and relies on records made routinely or as part of specific clinical studies. This information on the earlier period provides a less than complete set of data for our purposes. For the period 1982 to September 1984 our own data is more reliable and comprehensive and it is on data from this period that most of this Chapter is based.

With the inevitable focus of public attention on the number of actual transplants, the size of the underlying patient selection process tends to go unnoticed. Since the beginning of the current programmes, in 1979 at Papworth and 1980 at Harefield, a combined total in excess of 784 have been referred to the centres. Of those some 458 patients (or 58%) have been formally assessed. Of those assessed, approximately 68 per cent were initially "definitely accepted". (As a result of subsequent reclassification this percentage rose to 72 per cent.) At 30th September 1984, 221 patients had been transplanted, and of these patients seven had gone on to receive a second or "retransplant". In addition at that date there were 32 definitely accepted patients awaiting transplant.

TABLE 2.2 shows the total size of the programmes since their inception at the two centres and the allocation of assessed and non-assessed patients into various sub-groups. The problem in presenting such figures is that reassessment occurs and patients may be transferred to a different sub-group from that to which they were initially allocated. TABLE 2.3 illustrates the more complex picture that emerges once transfers between categories are taken into account. It shows, just for definitely accepted patients, the transfers in and out of the category as patients are reassigned.

2.4 The referred population

The data on the patients referred between January 1982 and September 1984 is summarised in TABLE 2.4 which gives breakdowns by age, sex, diagnosis, source of referral and country of residence. FIGURE 2.5 indicates the geographical distribution of patients' residence.

The following points (based on the combined Harefield and Papworth figures) perhaps deserve highlighting:
* The sex ratio of referrals was 6.9:1 (male:female).
* The vast majority of referrals are secondary referrals from hospital doctors. A small and decreasing number come from General Practitioners.
* Forty-two per cent of patients referred were within the age range 45–54 years and a further 27 per cent in the range 35–44 years.
* Ischaemic heart disease is the most common diagnosis (51% of referrals); cardiomyopathy is the next most common (36%).
* The Centres serve a geographically very wide catchment area which includes the whole of England, Wales and Scotland and patients' home towns are widely dispersed.

13

Table 2.2   The referrals to the two programmes + (as at 30 September 1984)

	Harefield	Papworth
Referrals:	324 *	460**
Assessed:*** Total	217 + +	241 + +
of which *initially*:		
Definitely accepted	183	130
Provisionally accepted	8	41
Offered other operation	10	31
Unsuitable for transplant	16	39
Died during assessment	22	3
Not assessed: Total	87	216
of which:		
Current referrals (awaiting decision whether to assess or not)	17	9
Died before decision to admit or not	16	2
Rejected at referral	27	170
Died before admission for assessment	13	25
Undergoing assessment	0	2
Declined offer of assessment	8	8
Referred: No further contact	4	—

+ All figures in this TABLE relate to numbers of patients — a small number of patients will have been assessed more than once.

+ + Includes a small number of patients assessed out of the two centres.

* All referrals from January 1982 onwards but only partial figures for non-assessed referrals for previous years.

** First three patients were referred and assessed in 1977–1978.

*** Assessed: defined as those for whom assessment completed.

Table 2.3   The definitely accepted category (as at 30 September 1984)

	Harefield	Papworth
Definitely accepted category:		
As initial decision:	183*	130**
Transferred to:—Provisional	—	6
—Unsuitable	4	2
Transferred from:—Provisional	2	12
—Unsuitable	—	5
—from other operation	—	4 +
'Net' Total	181	143
of which:—Transplanted	135	86
—Died awaiting transplant	22	46
—Declined transplant	2	—
—Still waiting	21	11
—Transplanted elsewhere***	1	—

* Plus three patients reaccepted and retransplanted.

** Plus four patients reaccepted and retransplanted.

*** Patient transplanted at National Heart Hospital.

+ Four patients transplanted after initially receiving other operation.

Table 2.4 Characteristics of patients referred and of patients assessed (1 January 1982 – 30 September 1984)

	Harefield		Papworth	
	Referred	Assessed	Referred	Assessed
Total number:	250	158	230	140
Male:	217	144	199	120
Female:	33	14	27	20
Unknown:	—	—	`4	—
Age:				
24 years and under	22	11	16	11
25–34	22	12	35	21
35–44	54	39	76	55
45–54	113	80	87	53
55 and over	37	16	14	—
Unknown	2	—	2	—
Diagnosis:				
IHD	142	93	105	69
CM	77	48	96	58
Other	31	17	25	13
Unknown	—	—	4	—
Referral:				
Hospital Doctor	231	152	215	135
General Practitioners	12	5	8	4
Non-medical	7	1	7	1
Residence:				
UK	201	127	213	140
Non UK	49	31	17	—

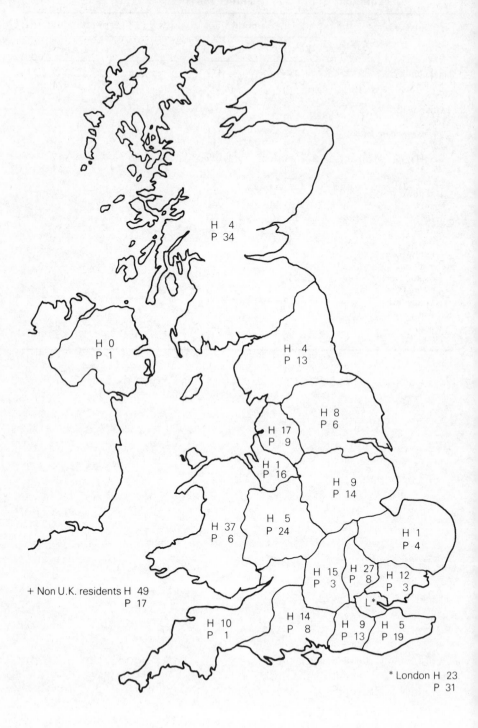

H 4
P 34

H 0
P 1

H 4
P 13

H 8
P 6

H 17
P 9

H 1
P 16

H 9
P 14

H 5
P 24

H 37
P 6

H 1
P 4

H 15
P 3

H 27
P 8

H 12
P 3

+ Non U.K. residents H 49
                   P 17

L *

H 10
P 1

H 14
P 8

H 9
P 13

H 5
P 19

* London H 23
         P 31

2.5 The assessment population

TABLE 2.4 indicates that the assessment population has very similar characteristics to the referred population from which it is drawn. The predominance of males is even more marked (7.8:1). The age dispersion is somewhat more compressed, although it may be noted that 10 per cent of patients assessed at Harefield were 55 or over. The breakdown of diagnoses between IHD and CM is very similar to that of the referred population. There is also a similarly wide geographical dispersion of patients' residence, as shown in FIGURE 2.6.

2.6 Transplant recipients

TABLE 2.7 summarises the characteristics of those who have received transplants in the period 1st January 1982 to 30th September 1984, and FIGURE 2.8 shows their geographical distribution. Not surprisingly, many of their characteristics are again similar to those of the referral population from which they are selected:

* The male predominance is even more marked than in the referred population. The male:female ratio amongst transplant recipients is 14.4:1 overall. However the ratios at the two centres are rather different: at Harefield the ratio is 17.3:1, whilst at Papworth a greater proportion of women have been transplanted with a ratio of 10.8:1.

* The age distribution is still more peaked: 46 per cent of patients were in the age range 45−54 years and 31 per cent in the range 35−44 years. It is notable again however that 8 per cent of transplant patients at Harefield have been 55 years or over, and further disaggregation of the age categories shows that 38 of Harefield's transplant patients (28%) were over the age of 50.

* The pattern of diagnoses is rather different between the centres. At Harefield 62 per cent are IHD patients and 31 per cent CM. At Papworth the split is rather more even — 51 per cent IHD and 41 per cent CM. This in part is reflected in the different age distributions (see Chapter Eleven).

* Twenty-two per cent of patients overall had undergone previous cardiac surgery — mainly coronary artery by-pass grafts. The proportion of previous cardiac surgery patients is considerably higher at Papworth (36%) than at Harefield (15%).

* The geographical dispersion is again very wide with patients coming from all but one of the English NHS Regions, Wales and Scotland, and in the case of Harefield from overseas.

2.7 The donor population

The other relevant population is that of the donors. TABLE 2.9 summarises the information for all donor hearts used at each centre, and FIGURE 2.10 indicates the geographical distribution of the hospitals from which the donor hearts were obtained. Predominantly in both centres the donors were young males under the age of 25 (63%). Most had died of cerebral trauma, frequently in road traffic accidents. At Harefield a rather higher proportion of female donors was used (28%) as compared to Papworth (14%). In 97 per cent of cases the kidneys were also removed for transplantation, and in several cases other organs were also utilised.

In addition to those used, many more hearts were offered. TABLE 2.11 shows

**Figure 2.6: Residence of patients assessed
(1 January 1982 - 30 September 1984)**

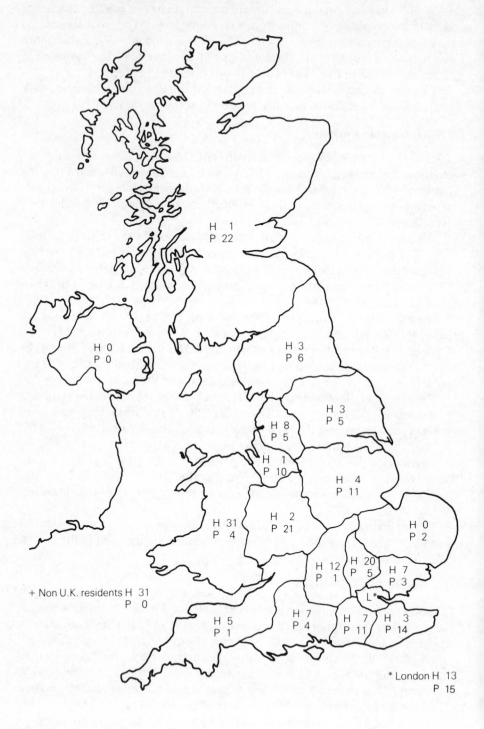

H 1
P 22

H 0
P 0

H 3
P 6

H 3
P 5

H 8
P 5

H 1
P 10

H 4
P 11

H 31
P 4

H 2
P 21

H 0
P 2

H 12
P 1

H 20
P 5

H 7
P 3

L *

+ Non U.K. residents H 31
P 0

H 5
P 1

H 7
P 4

H 7
P 11

H 3
P 14

* London H 13
P 15

18

Table 2.7   Characteristics of transplant recipients (1st January 1982–30th September 1984)

	Harefield	Papworth
Total Number:	110	59
Male	104	54
Female	6	5
Age:		
24 years and under	5	4
25–34 years	11	10
35–44 years	27	25
45–54 years	58	20
55 years and over	9	—
Diagnosis:		
IHD	68	30
CM	34	24
VHD	6	4
Other	2	1
Duration of illness:		
6 months and under	18	8
6–12 months	9	6
1–5 years	57	28
6–10 years	21	11
10 years and over	11	6
Number of Myocardial Infarctions:		
None	42	27
1	24	19
2 or more	44	13
Previous cardiac surgery:		
Patients	16	21
Operations	20	25
Types of Surgery:		
CABG	12	17
Other	9	13

**Figure 2.8: Residence of patients who have received transplants
(1 January 1982 - 30 September 1984)**

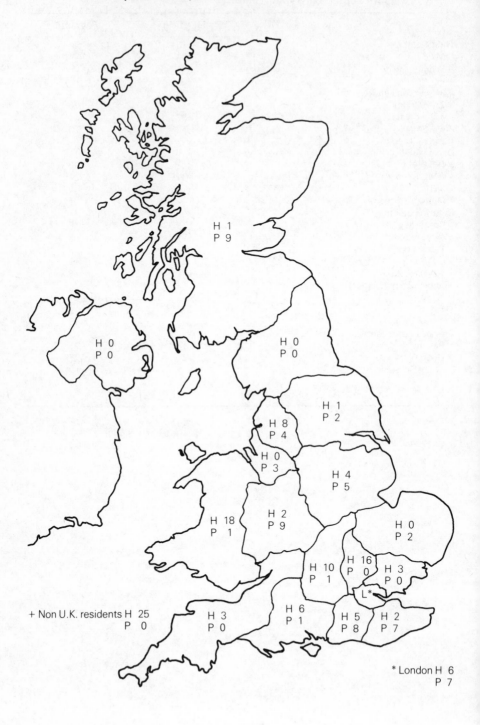

H 1
P 9

H 0
P 0

H 0
P 0

H 1
P 2

H 8
P 4

H 0
P 3

H 4
P 5

H 18
P 1

H 2
P 9

H 0
P 2

H 10
P 1

H 16
P 0

H 3
P 0

L*

+ Non U.K. residents H 25
P 0

H 3
P 0

H 6
P 1

H 5
P 8

H 2
P 7

* London H 6
P 7

20

Table 2.9   Donor hearts used (1st January 1982 – 30 September 1984)

	Harefield	Papworth
Total Number:	115	63
Male	83	54
Female	32	9
Age:		
24 years and under	72	40
25–34 years	29	15
35–44 years	14	7
45–54 years	0	1
Cause of death:		
Cerebral Trauma	75	47
Intracranial Haemorrhage	29	12
Respiratory Arrest	4	4
Cerebral Tumour	5	—
Others	2	—
Other Organs donated:		
Kidneys	112	61
Eyes	15	22
Liver	20	10
Pancreas	6	3
Skin	2	1
None	1	2

**Figure 2.10: Location of donor hospitals
(1 January 1982 - 30 September 1984)**

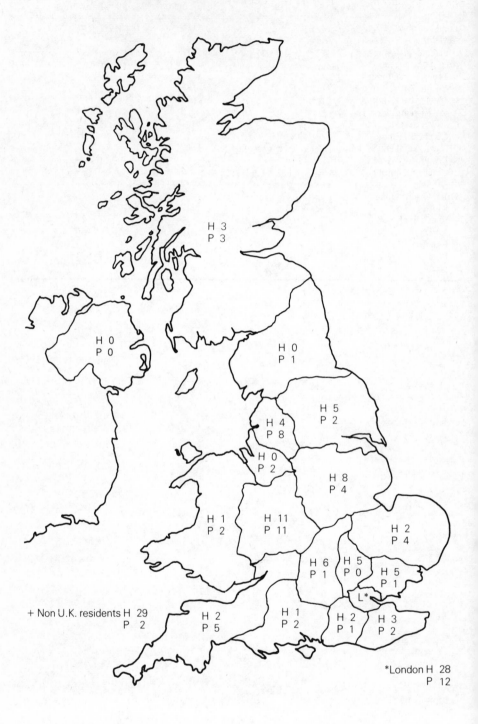

H 3
P 3

H 0
P 0

H 0
P 1

H 5
P 2

H 4
P 8

H 0
P 2

H 8
P 4

H 1
P 2

H 11
P 11

H 2
P 4

H 6
P 1

H 5
P 0

H 5
P 1

L*

+ Non U.K. residents H 29
P 2

H 2
P 5

H 1
P 2

H 2
P 1

H 3
P 2

*London H 28
P 12

22

Table 2.11 Reasons for non-use of offered donor hearts +

	Harefield*		Papworth		
	1983	1984 (to 30 Sept)	1982	1983	1984 (to 30 Sept)
Necessary resources not available	7	36	14	20	29
No suitable recipient	8	8	7	12	10
Organ/Donor unsuitable	6	34	14	21	28
Insufficient time to prepare	5	6	1	3	7
Consent/legal problems	7	6	4	5	4
Unknown	10	12	—	—	—
Total:	43	102	40	61	80

+ Organs may have been offered to both centres and appear in the figures for each.
* Data for 1982 not available.

the numbers offered but not used and the main reasons for non-use. The figures emphasise that it is not an overall shortage of suitable organs that currently limits the expansion of the programme. More frequently it is a limitation of available resources. Thus in the first nine months of 1984 at least 36 donor hearts were offered to Harefield and 29 to Papworth which, though suitable for a recipient, could not be used due to some form of resource constraint.

2.8 Summary

Although the programmes are complex, and subject to detailed differences between the centres, the two programmes are fundamentally similar involving a two-stage screening procedure to select patients, firstly using information available at referral and then if appropriate a detailed assessment usually carried out at the transplant centres. Specific patient selection criteria exist for each centre: the prime factor is the presence of imminently fatal heart disease which cannot be treated by further medical therapy or conventional surgery. Similarly criteria for donor suitability, and donor-recipient compatability have been spelt out.

For the whole period of the programmes since 1979 (and up to 30th September 1984), a combined total in excess of 784 patients had been referred. Of these 58 per cent had been assessed, and around 70 per cent of those assessed were definitely accepted for transplantation. At 30th September 1984, 221 patients had received transplants.

We have recorded data on the age, sex and diagnosis of all patients referred, assessed, and transplanted since 1st January 1982. The vast majority (93%) who have received transplants are male. There are two main diagnoses: fifty-eight per cent suffered from ischaemic heart disease and 34 per cent from cardiomyopathy. The biggest group of patients were in the 45–50 year age group, although the age distribution for cardiomyopathy patients was lower than for IHD patients. The Papworth surgeons do not normally accept patients over the age of 50 years but at Harefield the normal age limit is 59. Just over 20 per cent of transplant patients had undergone previous cardiac surgery.

Patients are drawn from a very wide geographical area and residents from all the English NHS Regions and of Scotland and Wales have been assessed.

The donor organs come principally from young males under the age of 25, who have died of cerebral trauma, frequently in road traffic accidents. In almost all cases the kidneys were also removed for transplantation. Particularly in 1984, many suitable donor hearts have been offered but could not be used because the necessary resources were not available to carry out further transplants at the particular time.

3. Levels of Activity, Lengths of Stay, and Bed Use

3.1 Introduction

Before analysing in detail the costs of the programmes, it may help to indicate some broader parameters (related to cost) that give some indication of the overall demands made by the programme in terms of the changing level of activity at the two centres, of the changes in the length of stay at the different stages in the programme, and of the resultant overall impatient bed usage.

From the point of view of the impact of the programme on the two centres, the figures for overall bed-usage provide an important indicator, particularly if the availability of staffed beds is a major constraint in the service, rather than say theatre time or support facilities. In terms of the desire to portray the experience of the "average" transplant patient, lengths of in-patient stay constitute a ready indicator, which can fairly easily be compared with equivalent figures for other types of operation, procedure or treatment.

It must be stressed however *that the figures in this Chapter relate only to activity in Harefield and Papworth,* and not to any work at other hospitals related to the care of the patients being studied.

3.2 Level of activity over time

At the commencement of the study it was expected that for the three years, if funding was available for that long, the level of activity would be approximately 15−20 transplants per annum at each centre. In the event the rate of transplantion at Papworth has been rather higher than this in 1984. At Harefield the number of transplants has been considerably higher than originally expected; up to end of September 1984 the number was already three times greater than for the whole of 1982. However, at Harefield the rate of new assessments is now little higher than the rate of transplant operations. (These figures intentionally exclude any assessments carried out elsewhere.) TABLE 3.1 sets out for Harefield and for Papworth the numbers of referrals, assessments, and transplant operations by year.

The impact of this workload is rather atypical in that organ availability makes the timing of the transplant operations upredictable. Most take place out of normal operating hours. This is clearly shown in TABLE 3.2, which uses an illustrative categorisation of time of day indicating that between January 1982 and September 1984 only a quarter of the combined number of transplants began in the "normal" hours of 0800 — 1800 on a week day. At Harefield a decreasing proportion now take place during that period (20% in 1984), whilst at Papworth there was considerable increase in 1984 to 32 per cent.

The predominance of "out of hours" work appears to reflect a number of factors:

25

Table 3.1 Levels of activity of the transplant programmes within the two centres over time

	1979 (and earlier)	1980	1981	1982	1983	1984 (to 30 Sept)
Harefield						
Referrals	4*	33*	37*	61	73	116
Assessments	4	28	27	36	37	62
Transplant operations	0	14	13	20	34	57
Papworth						
Referrals	43	145	54	77	63	78
Assessments	12	53	39	50	46	49
Transplant operations	3	11	13	16	19	28

* Incomplete records of unassessed referrals available prior to 1982

Table 3.2 Time of day of the commencement of transplant operations (January 1982 — September 1984)

	Monday — Friday			Saturday — Sunday			Total
	08.00–18.00	18.00–24.00	00.00–08.00	08.00–18.00	18.00–24.00	00.00–08.00	
	'In hours'			'Out of hours'			
Harefield							
1982	7	8	2	2	1	0	20
1983	12	11	3	7	1	0	34
1984	11	23	7	8	8	0	57
Papworth							
1982	2	10	1	2	1	0	16
1983	1	8	2	6	2	0	19
1984	9	10	2	4	3	0	28

(a) a conscious choice at both Centres to operate out of hours in an attempt to minimise the effect on planned theatre lists and schedules;

(b) the need to co-ordinate timing of the removal of the donor heart to follow immediately the removal of the kidneys by the renal team, who frequently themselves are time constrained for the reason noted as (a) above. (It will be remembered that in 97 per cent of donor operations the kidneys were also removed.)

(c) the externally imposed timing of the availability of a potentially suitable donor, itself an event which may well be biased towards out of hour times and weekends.

We have not been able to assess in detail the specific effect of this unusual pattern of working. In the earlier stages of the programme, with low transplantation rates, the effect may well have been to reduce the impact of the programme on the other work of the hospitals. This was made easier by goodwill and enthusiasm, and the willingness of the hospital staff generally to absorb much of the extra work through longer and unsocial hours and extraordinary effort.

We are aware that this goodwill has recently been stretched by the increasing activity levels, and that the ability of the resources of the two hospitals to absorb the extra workload required for transplantation as a non-integral addition to their "normal" workload is now in doubt.

The implication, as we see it, is that if the programmes are to continue they must become much more an integral and planned element of the overall "normal" workload of the hospitals. Inevitably the unpredictability of donor availability will mean for the foreseeable future that transplant activity cannot be planned in detail in advance, but it may be possible to plan more fully for the possibility of a transplant taking place, and certainly for the other elements of the work of the transplant programme. Indeed in the longer term, technical advances in the preservation of donor organs may increase the surgeons' ability to choose when to operate.

3.3. Lengths of stay

Figures on length of stay for the two centres, based on records for all the transplant patients in the relevant years (see TABLE 3.1), reveal rather different patterns of hospitalisation (TABLE 3.3).

At Papworth during the whole period of our study an essentially standardised assessment procedure has occurred and was organised so that it normally took place over three days. It relies on the patients having had various tests carried out in advance at their local hospital or referring centre. Thus the mean length of stay at assessment over the period 1 January 1982 — 30 September 1984 was 3.1 days, a figure that reflects a slight increase in the length of stay in each of the three years 1982 to 1984. [The yearly figures were 2.7, 3.2 and 3.4 respectively.]

At Harefield the mean length of stay for assessments has fallen dramatically from a figure on 17.3 days in 1982 to 8.9 days in 1984, although this figure is still considerably greater than that for Papworth. This reflects, amongst other factors, much less reliance than at Papworth on the carrying out of tests else-where in advance of admission.

Table 3.3 Average lengths of inpatient stay at various treatment stages (1 January 1982 — 30 September 1984)

	1982	1983	1984 (to 30 Sept)	1982–1984
Harefield				
Assessment	17.3	9.9	8.9	11.3
Period between assessment and transplant	8.7	3.8	1.7	4.1
Transplant to discharge	30.3	18.0	13.2	17.6
Post discharge stay in flats	20.5	13.7	12.4	14.2
Transplant to death (prior to discharge)	20.6	22.5	12.0	16.9
Papworth				
Assessment	2.7	3.2	3.4	3.1
Period between assessment and transplant	0.3	0.3	0.1	0.2
Transplant to discharge	51.9	46.1	44.4	46.8
Post discharge stay in village	0	0.3	1.5	0.7
Transplant to death (prior to discharge)	17.4	21.0	16.8	17.5

A declining but still significant proportion of patients spend some time in the centre between assessment and transplant. Some of these are readmissions, due to deterioration in the health of the patient, others are admitted for an expected transplant that does not in the end happen and a "false-start" preparation occurs. In addition, particularly at Harefield, patients too ill to be sent home tended to "wait" as inpatients until a transplant was possible. The figures for this period between assessment and transplant show a considerable decline at Harefield from 8.7 days in 1982 to 1.7 days in 1984. At Papworth they have never been significant: 0.3 days in 1982, 0.3 days in 1983 and 0.1 days in 1984.

The figures for postoperative lengths of stay are rather different. At both Centres duration has been falling, but there remains a substantial difference between the two Centres for the lengths of inpatient stay for patients discharged alive during the period from 1 January 1982. The figures for 1984 for this post-operative period as inpatients are 13.2 days at Harefield and 44.4 days at Papworth. Some of this difference is explained by the use of the "transplant flats" provided in Harefield village by the Harefield Heart Transplant Trust, which provide a "half-way-house" for many patients between their being discharged as an inpatient and their actual return home if it is some distance away from the Centre. During this period in the flats, they can attend Harefield Hospital regularly (initially daily) as out-patients. Recently an arrangement was made for three Papworth patients, who lived far away, to be discharged to accommodation in the village of Papworth for a few days. If this period, currently averaging 12.4 days at Harefield but averaging out to only 1.5 days at Papworth, is added in, the average overall postoperative length of stays prior to discharged home are 25.6 days at Harefield and 45.9 at Papworth. Separate average lengths of post transplant IP stay are shown for those who died prior to discharge: 12.0 days at Harefield and 16.8 at Papworth in 1984.

The frequency of readmissions is extremely difficult to present in terms of averages per patient but is included in the figures in the next section (3.4) and is dealt with in some detail in Chapter Seven.

3.4 Bed use — inpatient days

TABLE 3.4 summarises the total number of in-patient bed-days used by patients on the transplant programme at each centre. The figures for the thirty-three month period to 30 September 1984 show a total of 5,226 days at Harefield and 3,995 days at Papworth. During this period it will be remembered, 111 cardiac transplantations were performed at Harefield and 63 at Papworth thus the two sets of bed-use figures reflect different levels of transplant activity during the relevant period. These figures and the annual figures they summarise give one indication of the overall impact of the programmes on the resources of the hospitals. What should be noted however from the detailed breakdown is that the bed-usage by patients between their operations and discharge (or death in hospital prior to discharge) is but part of the total demand made by the programme. This period of immediate post-transplant care accounts for only 37 per cent of the total demand for beds made by the programme at Harefield and 66 per cent at Papworth. Whilst these two proportions are very different from each other, both clearly indicate the importance of the parts of the programme other than the immediate postoperative period.

28

Table 3.4   Bed usage by patients in the transplant programme (1 January 1982 — 30 September 1984)

Number of inpatient days	1982	1983	1984 (to 30 Sept)	1982–1984
Harefield				
Assessment	602	452	545	1599
Period between assessment and transplant	292	156	134	582
Posttransplant care to discharge or death in hospital	558	622	745	1925
Postoperative readmissions	257	352	511	1120
Total	1709	1582	1935	5226
Papworth				
Assessment	136	145	164	445
Period between assessment and transplant	16	15	3	34
Posttransplant care to discharge or death in hospital	886	817	927	2630
Postoperative readmissions	252	360	274	886
Total	1290	1337	1368	3995

3.5 Summary

The annual numbers of transplant operations has increased considerably over the last three years. For Papworth the figure of 28 transplant operations during the first nine months of 1984 was 75 per cent higher than the figure for the whole of 1982; for Harefield the comparable figure of 57 transplant operations was an increase of 85 per cent. In addition a significantly larger number of patients are assessed each year.

For a number of reasons, a large proportion of the operations take place out of "normal" operating hours — in the evenings, at night or at the weekends. The ability of the staff of the hospitals to continue to absorb this transplant activity as a net addition to their workload is now in doubt.

At Papworth the average length of stay at assessment has remained fairly constant at just over three days. The length of stay from transplant operation to discharge has fallen somewhat and the average for 1984 is 44.4 days.

At Harefield the length of stay at assessment has almost halved but is still just under nine days. The fall in length of postoperative stay is even more dramatic and this is now down to 13.2 days, plus an average of 12.4 days post discharge stay in one of the flats provided for the use of transplant patients in Harefield village.

The overall usage of beds within the hospitals for the two programmes as a whole in the first nine months of 1984 was in the order of 1,935 bed-days at Harefield and 1,368 bed-days at Papworth.

4. Costing Concepts

4.1 Introduction

The remit of the study included the consideration of two aspects of cost: (a) "the analysis of all resource costs within Papworth and Harefield Hospitals associated with their respective programmes"; and (b) "the identification and analysis of extra costs to the NHS and other parts of the public sector incurred outside the two centres by the patients involved in the transplant programmes and their selection procedures".

The first of these is conceptually simple although in practice not without difficulty given the inadequacy for such purposes of the routine hospital costing systems. The second element, focussing on the *extra* costs presents problems of a more conceptual nature in that it involves, in the absence of a formal control group, the estimation of what might otherwise have been the costs incurred in caring for patients who entered into the transplant programmes. This Chapter sets out the costing concepts and principles we have adopted.

4.2 Costs incurred within Harefield and Papworth Hospitals

Our analysis attempts throughout to measure and value resources used rather than financial flows as such. Nevertheless, *in general* we have to rely on the prices paid as indicators of the opportunity cost value of the resources used. In the present context, it is important to stress that the costs we identify are not conceptually the same as the extra funding that the two hospitals have needed to provide the programmes. For example, some resources that existed prior to the establishment of the programmes may now be being used more efficiently and fully; similarly, other resources provided as a result of the programmes may be used to the benefit of other patients. Our approach has been to estimate "average unit costs" for particular resources or services which "spread" the total cost of that resource or service over its total patient usage. Thus if the same costing procedures, as those we are applying to transplant patients, were applied to all other categories of patients treated within each of the Centres, the value of the total resources involved would be accounted for. This means that our figures generally can be related closely to those in the hospital cost statements. Instances where different and more appropriate conventions have been adopted are noted. (For convenience we include but identify separately within our analysis of the in-centre hospital costs the costs of certain resources not normally paid for out of local NHS funds. Examples are the cost of the hospital social worker and the full cost of blood-products supplied by the transfusion service.)

It is tempting to argue that each programme should be costed in terms of just short-run marginal costs; that is to say in terms of the immediate increase in resources consumed by the hospital as a result of the introduction of the programme. Many general administrative, support and technical services, and other

30

overheads might appear to be unaffected by marginal increases in the overall levels of hospital activity, resulting from the introduction of the programme. Hence short-run marginal costs in these areas might be negligible. However in terms of decisions concerning the longer-term, an average cost including an overhead element is more appropriate, because it reflects the fact that in the longer-run the scale of almost all activities and support services can be adjusted to reflect the total level of workload within the hospitals.

Such an "all-inclusive" average cost is perhaps most useful in the context of planning decisions, where a service development is being considered, of which an integral part would be a programme of cardiac transplantation. Central decisions about the long-term development of heart-transplantation need to consider the total costs of programmes in the future, and hence need to consider average rather than marginal costs per patient.

However in a different decision context, where for example the question is whether or not to increase the size of an existing programme, it is likely that some existing resources previously not fully utilised will be used more fully and others, already fully utilised, will be partially diverted from other uses. In such a situation certain average costs may be overestimates of the financial impact of the programme.

More generally, it is hazardous to extrapolate the costs of an essentially innovatory programme to those that would be incurred by a routine and accepted service.

On the one hand, at the early "experimental" stage of such programmes, extra costs may be incurred. Understandable caution may lead to the use of what subsequently turns out to be unnecessarily high levels of nursing, or use of tests, that in future, as experience is gained, can be reduced. As might be inferred from the data in Chapter Three on lengths of stay, many aspects of cost have been falling during the course of the programmes. In Chapters Six and Seven we present the costs so that this decline can be observed. Where trends are emerging, it seems reasonable to plan for the future on the basis of extrapolations of more recent experience.

On the other hand, "innovatory" situations may produce lower costs. Both the programmes that we have been observing have been facilitated by the willingness of staff to absorb much of the extra work through longer and (unsocial) hours and extraordinary effort. Clinicians have been at pains to ensure that their normal workload was not affected. It seems inevitable that as, and if, such programmes become routinely accepted they would tend to attract less extraordinary support from staff and have to be treated much more as an integral element of normal workload. Thus for example, whilst in the short-run it may be possible to argue that actual staff hours involved should be treated as affecting overtime levels at the margin, it is more reasonable to assume that in the longer-term appropriate adjustments would be made to the establishment of all the staff groups affected. It is clear that such pressures are now being felt in both Centres.

Furthermore it should be noted that in attempting to identify and measure actual resources used, we make no judgement as to the necessity or effectiveness of their use. It is true that the funding arrangements for the projects have made the clinicians more than usually cost-conscious. Indeed the experience with the transplant programme "budgets" perhaps offers some general pointers to the potential value of specialty or sub-specialty budgeting. We know that the exist-

31

ence of the project has made staff at the two Centres more aware of differences in the practices between them, and has led them in some instances to question and to adjust their behaviour. This has been, we believe, an important positive side-effect of the research.

We suspect our presence and the data we have collected have led directly to some changes in behaviour, but we have nevertheless attempted simply to record what resources are used, and have not attempted to make judgements about how things *might* better be organised. Thus the costs of the programmes are intended to reflect the *actual* efficiency of resource usage of the various hospital departments concerned, rather than some theoretical concept of what ought to be achievable.

To put the issue in a rather different way, the levels of resources used in nursing, for example, may reflect the levels of resources available rather than some independent concept of resources needed. The cost figures we quote represent neither ideals nor targets; no more are they minima or for that matter maxima. They simply relate to the actual situation in the two hospitals, not to some theoretical construct.

Finally, we have tried to distinguish between the costs that should correctly be attributed to the provision of the transplantation programme as a service activity and those attributable to related research. In practice the dividing line is often hard to draw. Where costs are undoubtedly concerned only with research we have not included them. Where the dividing line is less clear cut we have attempted to show them as separate items. However given that we are evaluating the programme in terms of its service benefits only, it is important to measure only the costs relating to that service and not to research. The costs and benefits of the research activities are a separate issue.

4.3 Costs incurred elsewhere

The boundary between "in centre" and "out of centre" costs is important yet artificial. It is important in that only the "in-centre" costs are normally considered part of the costs of the programmes — and a possible claim on non-local funds. Yet the boundary reflects particular practice and can be shifted as a deliberate policy decision. Given the way that funds are allocated, such shifts are of considerable importance to the hospitals concerned. They are much less important to the NHS as a whole. For example, ensuring that certain tests are carried out on patients at the referring centre prior to assessment reduces the transplant centre's costs with respect to that patient. However the costs to the NHS as a whole may be lower or higher depending upon the costs of the local hospital relative to those of the transplant centre. For this reason, if for none other, cost comparisons between the two centres have to be made with the utmost caution.

We have attempted to identify the extra resources used elsewhere in the NHS as a result of the referral and assessment process, in the period between assessment and transplant, and post discharge, using information from interviews, diaries kept by the patients, and a survey of referring consultants. These costs are discussed in Chapter Seven.

4.4 Capital costs

All the preceeding discussion of costs, like so much costing in the NHS, is concerned only with revenue or running costs. In the absence of any formal capital accounting system the estimation of capital costs, however theoretically valid it may be, is not only difficult but of questionable practical relevance.

In neither Centre is there a significant and definable element of capital stock (be it buildings or major equipment) that constitutes the "transplant centre" devoted solely to use by the transplant programme. The vast majority of capital resources used are simply those available to patients in the hospital as a whole, or more particularly those used by cardiac surgery patients as a whole. Particular capital spending nominally related to the transplant programmes during the period in question gives little indication of the actual claim on capital resources.

We therefore report on two aspects of capital cost. Firstly, we have calculated an average capital cost per inpatient day. This is based on a detailed capital costing of a theoretical DGH which has been carried out by the Works Group at the DHSS [DHSS, 1981]. The detail of this calculation is reported in the next chapter.

Secondly, we have identified specific expenditures on equipment and building, that have been seen as relating to the transplant programmes. These items are simply indicative of the additional capital spending that has been incurred at the two hospitals given their existing cardiac surgery and other facilities.

Unfortunately we have not been able to calculate a capital cost for each use of specific equipment. Such a calculation would require much more detailed information than is available to us on, for example, levels of usage and the equipment's length of service life.

4.5 Summary

The focus of our analysis of costs is the value of resources used rather than financial flows. Although prices paid are usually the best available indicators of opportunity costs, conceptually the costs so identified are not necessarily the same as the extra funding received by the two hospitals. The approach we have adopted has been to estimate " average unit costs" for particular resources or services used in the programme.

The levels of resources used may reflect the levels available rather than an independent concept of those ideally needed. Thus our figures are not targets, nor maxima, nor minima. They simply reflect the actual levels of resources used by the programme during the period of study. In accordance with the treatment of benefits, we have endeavoured to cost only the patient service element and to exclude research costs.

Because the two centres differ considerably in the extent to which they rely on tests etc undertaken elsewhere, comparison between them has to be made with extreme caution. Such external costs have been estimated on the basis of patients' diaries, interviews and a survey of referring consultants.

No definable element of capital stock belongs solely to the transplantation programme (or "centre") in either hospital. Whilst specific capital spending associated with the development of the programmes can give some indication of the sorts of costs that might be incurred elsewhere, depending upon their existing resources, a theoretical "full" capital cost per inpatient day provides a better baseline indicator of the overall cost of capital used.

5. Costing Methodologies and Conventions

5.1 Introduction

This chapter deals with the details of the sources of information about each of the main resources used by the programmes and on the unit costs calculated for them. There is no unique solution to the problem of how best to estimate costs. Our approach for any particular item involves a series of detailed assumptions and conventions. We have endeavoured to make these consistent between the two centres: any major divergencies of approach have been noted. However, differences between the centres in the cost of individual elements may reflect different organisational arrangements rather than substantive differences in the resources used. For example, figures for Harefield include London Allowance within staff costs where appropriate. Comparisons are further obscured by the differing degrees of support and interrelationship of services provided by each Centre from and to neighbouring hospitals. Harefield looks to Mount Vernon Hospital close by for some support services; other services are provided on a combined or even district-wide basis. Papworth has close ties with Addenbrooke's Hospital in Cambridge for certain specialist services, but also has organisational links with Hinchingbrooke Hospital, Huntingdon.

We would emphasise that our cost figures should not be used directly for detailed allocations to different departments. To calculate accurate unit costs for all services used would have involved us in detailed work-study exercises in all departments, and involved them in maintaining detailed records relating to workload and time spent. We have had to rely on cruder estimations in some cases, particularly where it is clear that the particular costs constitute only a small part of the total costs of the transplant programmes. Our estimates should however be indicative of the overall magnitude of short-run average costs, and the way these are built up from the various constituent resources used. (All costs are presented in terms of financial year 1983–84, or approximately September/October 1983.)

5.2 Costs of the time of the transplant surgeons

Four very detailed studies have been carried out at Papworth of the time allocation of the members of the surgical team (including the three consultant surgeons involved and their junior staff). In each study, the surgeons were surveyed over an eight-week period on seven separate days which constituted a cycle of one week. Detailed breakdowns of the way their total working time was allocated were obtained identifying patient care, administration, research, and teaching/conferences. Each of these categories was further split into transplant and non-transplant work. The results of the four studies are summarised in TABLE 5.1 with the figures expressed in terms of percent of whole time equivalents (wte's). There were some considerable differences between the first three studies in the pattern of time spent on the transplant programmes. The third and fourth studies were very similar.

The figures for the consultants at Papworth average to 112 per cent of a whole time equivalent spent on transplant work, split between patient care (59%), administration (2%), and research/teaching/conferences (51%). The relatively high percentage of time spent on research reflects in particular the joint NHS/British Heart Foundation research appointment held by one of the consultants concerned. For the junior doctors, the bulk of whose time with respect to the transplant programme is spent on direct patient care, the four studies produced an average allocation of time approximately equivalent to 90 per cent of a wte to the transplant programme as a whole, or 86 per cent to transplant patient care.

Table 5.1   Surgical staff time: Time allocated to transplant work as percentage of a whole time equivalent member of staff

	Study 1	Study 2	Study 3	Study 4	Average
Papworth					
Consultant Staff					
Patient care	82.7	39.6	57.1	57.5	59.2
Administration	2.6	6.2	0	0.7	2.4
Research/Teaching	57.3	84.2	32.2	28.2	50.5
Total	142.6	130.0	89.3	86.4	112.1
Junior Medical Staff					
Patient care	59.2	83.1	90.8	111.2	86.1
Administration	0	0	0	0	0
Research/Teaching	0	11.9	1.6	0	3.4
Total	59.2	95.0	92.4	111.2	89.5
Harefield					
Consultant Staff					
Patient care	14.2	13.4	27.0		18.2
Administration	0.6	4.4	4.4		3.1
Research/Teaching	0	0	0		0
Total	14.8	17.8	31.4		21.3
Junior Medical Staff					
Patient care	170.0	105.4	145.7		140.4
Administration	22.9	0	9.7		10.9
Research/Teaching	7.1	4.7	6.5		6.1
Total	200.0	110.1	161.9		157.4

At Harefield three surveys of the time of the consultant surgeon and his support staff have been carried out to obtain comparable information. These indicate that the programme as a whole accounts for 21 per cent of a consultant wte. This average reflects an increasing proportion of his time devoted to transplant work as the size of the Harefield programme has grown. Over the period of our research he has had a variety of different arrangements for support from junior

35

staff — and these are reflected in the three studies. At the time of the first study he was supported by two "transplant officers" of registrar status, who between them provided full cover for transplant patients, and 100 per cent of their time was devoted to transplant patient care and to research. In the second study the equivalent provision was provided by a clinical assistant, with night/weekend cover provided by the existing on call registrar or senior registrar from his cardiothoracic firm. This gave a somewhat lower cost than that of the previous arrangement. The third study reflected a period during which he had one transplant officer (who spent the majority of her time on transplant work) with the remaining support provided as part of the work of his firm. On average the three Harefield studies indicate an allocation of junior hospital doctors' time equivalent to 157 per cent of a wte. (This average matches closely the actual figures from the last study.)

For the main purposes of our evaluation we believe that it is inappropriate to include the cost of the time spent on research. The benefits of the programme are being assessed in terms of direct patient benefit and research benefits are not considered. The relevant cost figures should therefore be those of patient care and related administration. Certainly for the foreseeable future the programmes are likely to include a "research and development" element and the costs (and benefits) of this have to be considered, *even* if they are not met from NHS funds. But for our study, research costs should be excluded.

We have not been able to allocate surgical staff-time to specific patients. To do so would have required continuous record-keeping of doctor-patient contact times. Therefore these costs are treated as an "overhead" to the entire programme, and costed as a lump sum. Indeed, for the purposes of planning it may be conceptually more appropriate to consider the necessary surgical staff resources as an overhead to the programme. Costs have been based on the relevant total cost to the employing authority. The total costs are set out in TABLE 5.2. This shows a lump sum estimate of the costs per annum for the surgical staff time of £38 thousand at Harefield and £35 thousand at Papworth for transplant patient care and related administration (but excluding research).

5.3 Other medical staff

The *regular* use of time of other medical staff has however been included on a patient specific basis of an all inclusive cost per worked hour. For consultant staff the figures are £14.9 at Harefield and £14.0 at Papworth. We have costed in the subsequent chapters the routine use of a consultant psychiatrist to give a psychiatric report on patients at assessment; similarly for a consultant nephrologist at Harefield. In both Centres the time of anaesthetists at the transplant operation (and immediately before and after it) is specifically included in our costs per operation (summarised in Section 5.7 below). The time of the consultant pathologist is included in the costs of pathology services.

In addition, at Harefield alone, a significant number of patients undergo dental examination and treatment (to reduce the risks of infection at subsequent surgery). This treatment is provided by the hospital's dental department. We have related information on the number of transplant patients seen to the total work load and total costs of the dental service. Because of the considerable variability of the particular treatments provided we have not been able to cost by

Table 5.2 Annual programme costs of time of surgical teams

	Harefield	Papworth
	£	£
Patient care	34,392	34,572
Administration	3,428	788
Sub-total	37,820	35,360
Research	1,137	17,303
Total	38,957	52,663

patient, but have treated the cost (estimated at £4,450) as an overhead to the programme, principally to the assessment stage. For Papworth any such dental care is done at the patient's referring hospital or by a local dentist.

5.4 Nursing staff time

Much effort and time has been put into devising an appropriate method of measuring adequately the nursing input to the transplant programme that could be sensitive to the different demands made by patients of differing dependency and in nursing patients in differing locations.

The basic approach we adopted was to collect three main elements of relevant data:

(i) regular patient categorisation;

(ii) regular information on staffing levels;

(iii) sampled observation of nursing time related to patients in particular categories.

(i) *Patient Categorisation*

On the wards, we used Barr's patient categories (Barr [1964]). The categorisation into "self-care", "intermediate care" and "intensive care" has been carried out by the nursing staff using the detailed criteria as specified by Harper (Harper [1975] and Russell [1974]).

For intensive therapy units the same basic approach has been adopted but we have had to develop a specific ITU categorisation. Initially we adopted a four level categorisation which included an extra high care (crisis/emergency) category. This category proved to be applicable only as a transient state for patients, and when we attempted to time the care given to patients in this extreme category, it became clear that the state rarely lasted for even an hour of observation. It was therefore clearly inappropriate to distinguish it as a separate dependency state for the purposes of categorisation for a whole nursing. As a result the categorisation was collapsed to three states:

A - High Care

B - Medium Care

C - Low Care

The categorisation depends upon the patient's clinical condition/state in each of five body systems (cardio-vascular; respiratory; renal; nervous; and metabolic). The patients are allocated to whatever is the highest care state recorded for any of their body systems. The details of the categorisation of the patient's

Figure 5.3: I.T.U. NURSING DEPENDENCY CATEGORISATION

CARE GROUP A (HIGH DEPENDENCY)

CARDIOVASCULAR — cardiac instability or poor cardiac function: eg cardiac arrest; acute dysrhythmias; low or poor cardiac output (requiring mechanical support eg "balloon pump", or I.V. chemotherapy "supports"); heavy blood loss (over 150 mls/hr from drains).

RESPIRATORY failure or support:
eg failure leading to respiratory arrest; intubated and mechanically ventilated or being "tried off".

RENAL failure:
eg acute renal failure — requiring daily haemodialysis.

NEUROLOGICAL — deep coma — no reaction to painful stimuli and absent gag reflex; intra-cranial pressure monitoring (together with respiratory ventilation).

METABOLIC instability:
eg acute metabolic crisis — hepatic coma, diabetic coma;
liver failure leading to gastro-intestinal bleeding and mental confusion; gross electrolyte/acid imbalance.

CARE GROUP B (MEDIUM DEPENDENCY)

CARDIOVASCULAR — adequate cardiac state:
eg infrequent dysrhythmias; stable, chronic dysrhythmias; adequate cardiac output; minimal cardiac support (routine postoperative "supports" or weaning off other I.V. "supports"); moderate blood loss (80 mls/hr to 150 mls/hr from drains).

RESPIRATORY — self ventilation with some support:
eg extubated and requiring oxygen/humidification; may require nasopharyngeal suction; may have a tracheostomy.

RENAL — renal support in a steadily changing condition:
eg requires haemodialysis an alternate days or continuous peritoneal dialysis, or continuous haemo-filtration.

NEUROLOGICAL — deep coma — but pain response and gag reflex present;
intra-cranial pressure monitoring; gross confusion or mental irritation.

METABOLIC — impaired liver function:
eg ascites; portal hypertension; controlled diabetes (but still on sliding-scale insulin); close monitoring of electrolyte/acid base status.

CARE GROUP C (LOW DEPENDENCY)

CARDIOVASCULAR — stable cardiac function:
eg stable cardiac output; reducing, or no, cardiac support; minimal blood loss (less than 80 mls/hr.)

RESPIRATORY — self ventilation with minimal oxygen; may have tracheostomy.

RENAL — satisfactory renal function:
eg no longer requires dialysis; no inotropic support; may still be catheterised.

NEUROLOGICAL — drowsy but rousable; mild confusion.

METABOLIC — satisfactory liver function; controlled diabetes (not on sliding scale insulin), stable electrolyte/acid base status.

clinical condition for each of the five body systems is set out in FIGURE 5.3.

All patients in the ITUs and the wards mainly concerned with transplant patients ("E Ward" at Harefield and "Top Floor" at Papworth) have thus been categorised three times daily prior to the end of each shift on the basis of the patients' dependency at the time of changeover. This gives us a dependency profile throughout the inpatient period for all transplant patients since the autumn of 1982, as well as the patient information for the index of the overall workload on each of the relevant wards, and on the ITUs (see below).

(ii) Staffing Levels

At the same time as recording the patient dependency data, records have been made by the nurses of the numbers of the different grades of nursing staff available on the ward during each shift. This indicates the total nursing resources available.

(iii) Observational Timings

In addition over a period of months, sample timings of the observed direct nursing time spent with transplant and non-transplant patients in the different categories have been recorded to ascertain ratios of direct nursing time spent with patients of different dependency. The period covered has been 8:00am–8:00pm with an intended total of a minimum 100 hours per category (in blocks of one full hour) equally spread over the hours of the day, and equally distributed as far as possible between transplant and non-transplant patients. The number of hours of observation of ward care is shown on TABLE 5.4. The dividing line between ITU and Ward responsibility appears to be rather different at the two centres. There were rarely highly dependent (group 3) patients on the ward at Papworth because they were not normally transferred from ITU until they had progressed to the lower care group (group 2). At Harefield, patients rarely remained under ITU care if they had moved out of ITU Care Group B into C. From these observed timings, ratios of time spent with patients in different nursing dependencies can be calculated. TABLE 5.4 sets out the our timings at each Centre both for the wards and for ITU, and expresses them as mean averages for the direct nursing care provided per hour to each category of patient.

Before transforming these figures of direct nursing time into ratios, we applied tests of significant difference hierarchically between the observed timings for all patients in each care group (at each centre), and then between transplant and non-transplant patients within care groups. Only where statistically significant differences were found did we calculate separate ratios. Thus the same nursing time dependency ratios apply to transplant and non-transplant patients at Papworth in all but ITU Care Group A (the most intensive care). At Harefield higher ratios were found for the transplant patients in all but the least intensive category on the ITU and ward. The ratios are set out in TABLE 5.5.

There is a considerable overall similarity of the ratio scales between the two centres, although there are also obvious differences. It should perhaps be stressed that these differences between the centres reflect a variety of factors including staffing levels, relative availability of ward and ITU beds, and ward/ITU layout. It should also be emphasised that the "transplant" categorisation applies only to the post-transplant patients in the transplant rooms

Table 5.4 Sampled nurse timing (Ward and ITU) Minutes of direct nursing care per hour per patient

Harefield:

Care Group	Non Transplant Patients			Transplant Patients			All Patients		
	Mean (Minutes)	s.d.	No. of hours of observation	Mean (Minutes)	s.d.	No. of hours of observation	Mean (Minutes)	s.d.	No. of hours of observation
Ward 1	4.22	5.97	116	6.96	10.60	28	4.75	7.14	144
2	9.93	14.93	111	16.14	15.19	103	12.92	15.34	214
3	16.68	11.43	71	34.35	22.60	70	25.40	20.07	141
ITU C	28.31	9.78	14	43.47	—	1	29.32	10.20	15
B	42.20	16.94	95	65.51	18.83	90	53.54	17.85	185
A	58.59	15.05	100	72.79	15.09	131	66.64	15.07	231

Papworth:

Care Group	Non Transplant Patients			Transplant Patients			All Patients		
	Mean (Minutes)	s.d.	No. of hours of observation	Mean (Minutes)	s.d.	No. of hours of observation	Mean (Minutes)	s.d.	No. of hours of observation
Ward 1	2.79	3.73	60	3.53	5.05	43	3.10	4.33	103
2	5.05	5.39	72	5.56	13.33	30	5.20	8.46	102
3	32.94	30.58	16	—	—	0	32.94	30.58	16
ITU C	19.53	13.24	59	15.53	14.53	50	17.69	13.93	109
B	28.19	17.82	95	28.37	21.53	46	28.25	19.03	141
A	52.50	21.48	109	65.29	21.82	29	55.18	21.55	138

Table 5.5 Nursing Time Dependency Ratios: Harefield and Papworth

| | Harefield | | Papworth | |
	Transplant Patients	Non-Transplant Patients	Transplant Patients	Non-Transplant Patients
Nursing Dependency Care Group				
Ward: 1	1	1	1	1
2	3.4	2.1	1.7	1.7
3	7.2	3.5	10.6	10.6
ITU: C	6.2	6.2	5.7	5.7
B	13.8	8.9	9.1	9.1
A	15.3	12.3	21.1	16.9

at Harefield, or in ITU cubicles or single rooms on the ward at Papworth. Thus the higher timings may be as much a reflection of the effect of physical layout on nursing as of differences in actual patient dependency characteristics.

Using patient categorisation records and nurse staffing information for wards and ITU, these ratios have been applied as weights to construct a total work-load index against which to relate the actual available nursing hours per shift. These calculations are summarised in TABLE 5.6.

This analysis is based on the important assumption *that* total available nursing time (on ward or in ITU) can be allocated according to the Work Load index reflecting direct-nursing care timings. This crucial presumption that total care, including indirect care, is proportional to direct care is a common to most of this nursing dependency categorisation. Unfortunately it is an assumption that we have not been able to satisfactorily test.

Table 5.6 Nursing staff time: Hours per day* per workload unit

	Hours per workload unit +			Hours per patient
	Trained staff	Student/ course nurse	Aux. nurse	Ward clerk
Papworth:				
Ward	3.04	0.05	0.79	-
ITU	2.76	0.16	0.04	-
Harefield				
Ward	3.18	-	0.76	0.10
ITU	2.22	0.48	0.16	0.17

* Day is combination of observations made in three shifts; early, late and night, to give a twenty-four hour period.
+ The workload unit is equivalent to a patient in ward care group 1.

Finally, these hours of nursing time have been costed (at rates allowing for sickness absence, holidays, employers N.I. etc). From these nursing costs per day for each patient category have been calculated. These figures also include a nursing administration overhead to reflect the costs of senior nursing personnel not normally allocated to specific ward duties. These cost calculations are summarised in TABLE 5.7. There is a problem in deciding how most appropriately to deal with the costs of the student and course nurses. The costs of student (pupils) on the ward are not normally met by the hospital concerned. The cost of the "course nurses" (trained nurses undergoing specific cardio-thoracic training) are normally only charged in part to the hospital. Unit costs have been calculated both excluding and including the full cost of the student and course nurses, whose time contributions are separately identified in TABLE 5.6. From examination of the staffing levels and mixes on the wards and ITU it would appear that in the absence of either category of nurses, the numbers of other staff have to be increased, and we have therefore used the inclusive costs in our main costings. The costs of ward clerks are included in the "non-patient related" general services overhead (see Section 5.14).

In addition Harefield have allocated to a particular nurse, the specific responsibility for all out-patient visits by transplant patients. Her cost, which was £7716 in 1983–84, (based on the salary of an SRN plus on-costs, and nursing administration overhead) is again best seen as a specific overhead to the programme and has not been apportioned between patients.

5.5 Ward/ITU consumables

We experimented unsuccessfully with various alternative methods of attributing actual usage of consumables to specific patients, by detailed recording or by identifying and recording stores issued to specific wards, before deciding simply to apportion them. A priori there seems good reason to assume that the costs of these consumables is proportional to nursing dependency, and hence they have been calculated as fixed percentage of nursing costs. Our figure of 10 per cent of nursing costs is based on the sampled estimates of costs for the consumption of consumables in the ward and ITU at Harefield only. In each context, detailed costing of small samples produced cost figures that related very closely to those estimated by our 10 per cent "rule of thumb".

Table 5.7 Nursing costs per day per post operative transplant patient by dependency category

	Harefield		Papworth	
	Excluding course and pupil nurses	Including course and pupil nurses	Excluding course and pupil nurses	Including course and pupil nurses
	£	£	£	£
Patient Category:				
Ward: 1	18.8	18.8	17.9	18.0
2	63.9	63.9	30.4	30.6
3	135.4	135.4	189.7	190.8
ITU: C	74.4	89.9	78.7	83.2
B	165.6	200.1	125.6	132.9
A	183.6	221.9	291.2	308.1

Costs include an allowance for nursing administration but exclude costs of ward clerks. (The latter are included in the general administration overheads).

5.6 Drugs/Pharmacy

Drugs have been costed using detailed records of drugs provided for individual patients by Harefield and Papworth. The unit costs applied have been those that reflect local purchase prices allowing for discounts obtained, and adjusted where necessary to the September/October 1983 price base. Figures quoted include VAT, and a pharmacy "overhead" charge reflecting non-drug costs in pharmacy (essentially a "dispensing" cost). This "dispensing" add-on amounts to 15.0 per cent at Harefield and 10.5 per cent at Papworth.

Our costing of two particularly important drugs should be noted:

— the immunosuppressive drug Cyclosporin A, has been costed at the commercial price, although it was initally supplied for trial purposes free of charge.

— rabbit antithymocyte globulin (ATG), has in the past been supplied to Harefield non-commercially from Stanford University California, and its use in Harefield has been "costed" to reflect the voluntary contribution to Stanford for supplies provided. Supplies of equine ATG were provided to both Centres on a trial basis from a commercial supplier, although it now has a commercial market price. This price was used in the drug costings.

In costing the long-term care of transplant patients these same unit costs based on the two hospitals have been used for all drugs taken, including those obtained through GP prescription at dispensing chemists.

5.7 Costs of recipient operation

Patient specific data is available on the number and duration of transplant operations. The costs of the operation are an amalgamation of three basic elements.

(i) An average cost per transplant operation hour has been calculated for each hospital to reflect the staffing levels normal for a transplant operation. The transplant theatre time of surgical staff (who have *already* been included in the surgical time survey and costed as an overhead to the programmes) has of course been excluded from the staff cost per transplant operating hour to avoid double counting. Other medical time in theatre during transplantation, such as that of the anaesthetists, has been included in this cost per operating hour.

(ii) Our analysis of anaesthestists time also indicated the need to make a specific additional allowance for their significant input of time with the patient both immediately before and after the actual time of operation. Similar add-on allowances have been calculated based on estimates of the "extra" time of perfusionists, operating department staff, and an ECG technician as appropriate to each centre. These additional staff costs per transplant are shown in TABLE 5.8.

(iii) An average cost per operation has been estimated for non-staff items, including drugs, dressings and medical and surgical equipment used both generally and with the heart-lung (bypass) machine which is required in all transplant operations.

As TABLE 5.8 indicates, these cost elements are very similar at the two hospitals. The total cost per operation at Papworth is however significantly higher in that their transplant patients, unlike those at Harefield, are routinely fitted with pacemakers.

5.8 Respiratory physiology

Respiratory physiology tests (tests of lung-function and blood gases) have been

43

recorded for each patient. Such tests are carried out on the majority of assessment patients at Harefield, but were carried out on only five potential heart transplant patients at assessment at Papworth. We have calculated an average cost for each main type of test that reflects the relative time they take, apportioning the total departmental costs over the total estimated number of patient contact hours in the department. The figure so calculated for Harefield has been applied to the very few tests carried out on transplant patients at Papworth.

Table 5.8   Unit costs applicable to recipient operation

	Harefield £	Papworth £
Staff cost per transplant operating hour (excluding surgical staff)	84.9	66.9
Additional staff cost per transplant operation	149.1	116.3
Non-staff cost per transplant operation	278.2	296.8
Cost of pacemaker*	N/A	892.6

* Average cost allowing for reuse, after refurbishment, of 32 per cent of pacemakers.
N/A Not applicable to transplant patients at Harefield.

5.9 Radiography

Patient specific data have been collected on the frequency and type of investigations undertaken. National workload units are available for each procedure which represent the number of minutes of radiographers time taken in each procedure (DHSS [1972]). These overall measures of workload were originally calculated by means of actual procedure timings and expert professional judgement. Thus for costing purposes it is possible to use a department's annual recorded workload in units and relate this to total cost to derive a cost per workload unit and hence a cost per procedure. On this standard basis the cost per 100 units at Harefield is £23.64 and at Papworth is £36.04. In addition we have allowed within the costs of certain radiography procedures, for example, for the presence of an ECG technician.

However, the present system of measuring workload has a number of problems. Two particular criticisms that are of relevance to the transplant programmes are that (i) "a regular review to reflect technological advances particularly in the areas of ultrasound and CT, is needed" and (ii) "the additional weightings for the use of mobile/portable apparatus are in several cases excessive" (Whitt [1982]). Transplant patients undergo a number of increasingly sophisticated radiographical investigations for which national workload units are not readily available. In addition, transplant patients have a number of radiographic procedures on the ward or in the ITU, involving the use of portable equipment.

A sample survey, in which a limited number of procedures were timed, was undertaken at Papworth. No distinction was made between transplant and non-transplant patients. TABLE 5.9 indicates that the six procedures timed comprise approximately 72 per cent of the department's annual workload. Annual total units for each of the procedures was then weighted by the ratio of our timings to the prescribed national unit — thus producing an "adjusted total units" figure. Individual procedures were then costed according to their adjusted units as presented in TABLE 5.9. These observations suggest that with more accurate costing based on locally reweighted workload units, the range of the costs of the procedures most relevant to the heart transplant programme would be compressed. The low cost departmental X-rays would be increased in price and the high cost left-heart study considerably reduced.

However in the absence of a thorough reassessment of the whole workload of the departments at Papworth and at Harefield using O & M techniques, our main costings are all based on the "national" units.

Patients specific data on other less common "scans" has been costed. For some procedures, such as CT scanning, radiography workload units are available. For others, such as thallium, technetuim and gated blood pool scans, have been costed using sampled data on the average duration of the procedure in question and the costs of the professional and technical staff present. Because these scans are carried out outside Papworth, our unit costs are based on Harefield and applied to the data for Papworth as well.

Table 5.9   Papworth: Adjusted radiography units

Procedure	Prescribed units per procedure	Sample times (minutes) per procedure	Estimated annual units	Ratio of sampled times to units	Adjusted annual units	Cost per procedure (unadj. units) £	Cost per procedure (adj. units) £
Chest X-Ray							
— Department	6	8	41604	1.3	54085	2.2	6.3
— Ward	36	19	33804	0.5	16902	13.0	15.2
— ITU	66	44	158268	0.7	106039	23.8	36.1
Biopsy	90	29	30420	0.3	9734	32.4	23.8
Biopsy and right-heart catheter	180	93	4680	0.5	2386	64.8	76.4
Left-heart study	360	55	201960	0.2	30294	129.7	45.2
Total: Sampled procedures			470736		219440		
Total: All procedures			653166		304777		

5.10 Pathology

Pathology tests are ordered on request forms, and, although the number of tests per request form varies, records are normally kept only of the number of requests. An average ratio of tests per request form for all work coming to the pathology department in each of various main categories is routinely calculated on the basis of a small sample. (For details of the routine recording system see Ministry of Health [1963]). Our concern was that requests relating to transplant patients might be atypical in the number of tests they called for. Detailed studies have been undertaken by the research team of both centres, to establish transplant specific test/request ratios for each of the main elements of pathology. These enable us to use records of requests per patient as an accurate basis for costing. Separate ratios have been calculated for the preoperative, posttransplant inpatient, and postdischarge phases. Relating these to the average test/request ratios for the pathology departments, enabled us to calculate a cost per phase-specific transplant request, for biochemistry, microbiology, haematology and histology and to apply these to patient specific data. The transplant specific costs per request are presented in TABLE 5.10.

It should be emphasised that in comparing the figures in the two centres the differences in cost per request reflect a variety of factors including some differences in the amount of work per request as specified by the respective transplant teams. To cost more accurately would involve adopting a much more detailed method of establishing the costs of tests and recording all usage in terms of tests rather than requests. (A fuller discussion of the problems is given in Fabray [1983] and a possible detailed methodology in Stilwell [1981]).

Table 5.10   Estimated cost per transplant request for pathology tests

	Harefield	Papworth
	£	£
Bacteriology		
Preoperative	9.25	1.97
Operation to Discharge	6.25	1.81
Post discharge	6.62	1.62
Haematology		
Preoperative	2.74	1.66
Operation to Discharge	3.52	1.66
Post discharge	3.59	1.56
Chemical pathology		
Preoperative	12.41	2.39
Operation to discharge	8.47	2.39
Post disharge	8.89	2.98
Histology		
Preoperative		
Operation to Discharge ⎫	28.90	21.94
Post discharge ⎭		

Patient specific data have been collected on the frequency of T-cell tests and Cyclosporin assays. Normally all patients assessed and all donors are tissue typed; in addition all assessments have an anti-body screen. The two centres have different methods of organising these immunological tests.

Using the available information on technician time per Cyclosporin assay, consumables used and the number of patients tested in one assay, a cost per Patient assay of £4.7 has been calculated for Harefield. This figure has also been used in the costing for Papworth where the assays are carried out at Addenbrookes.

On a similar basis a cost per T-cell test (£14.6) has been calculated for Harefield and applied to both centres. Our cost of tissue typing (£50.0) is based on an estimate made by the tissue typing laboratory at Cambridge, and has been applied to the Harefield data. The cost of anti-body screening is included in the cost of haematology requests to the pathology labs for Harefield. It has been separately costed at an estimated £50.0 by the tissue typing laboratory who carry out the test for Papworth patients.

5.11 Electrocardiography

Records of the number of different types of tests carried out were maintained for each patient. Costs per test have been estimated based on information on the average time taken. These timings have been calculated as a proportion of the

46

Table 5.11   Electrocardiography: Cost per test

	Papworth		Harefield	
	assessment	Post transplant	assessment	Post transplant
	£	£	£	£
Department ECG	N/A	N/A	2.2	4.5
Portable ECG	1.2	2.4	3.0	6.7
Exercise ECG	N/A	N/A	11.8	11.8
24 Hour tape	N/A	N/A	24.3	24.3

N/A Not relevant to patients studied.

estimated total time spent by the departments in testing patients. This gives an average cost per test reflecting the total costs of the ECG departments (see Table 5.11).

Generally circumstances have been such that the demands of the programmes on the time of cardiologists have been minimised. Tests are normally read and assessed by the surgeons. However, reflecting current practice the cost of the time of a cardiology registrar is included in the cost of an exercise ECG at Harefield. Similarly an allowance for the time of a visiting consultant cardiologist, or of the consultant radiologist, at left-heart studies at Papworth has been added to the relevant unit radiography cost.

5.12 Blood products for transfusion

We have records of blood product usage by patient. These have been costed using the handling charges now applied to blood and blood derivatives supplied to non-NHS hospitals, as a measure of the full long-run marginal cost of supplying these items (DHSS [1984]). These costs do not include any element for the blood itself but do reflect the full costs of collection, processing, handling and transport. The charges, deflated back to October 1983 prices, are given in Table 5.12.

Table 5.12   Charges per unit for blood and blood derivatives used

	£
Whole blood	18.68
Plasma reduced blood/concentrated red cells	10.40
Platelet concentrate	10.40
Fresh frozen plasma (FFP)	10.40
Human plasma protein faction	33.10

5.13 Physiotherapy

Records of physiotherapists' time spent with specific patients have been collected. To these times we have applied an estimated average cost per patient contact hour for the physiotherapy services at each of the two centres. The figures reflect an estimate of the proportion of paid hours spent in patient contact which was based on discussions with the physiotherapists concerned.

5.14 General services

These are routinely divided into two standard categories: patient related services

47

Table 5.13   Annual programme costs of social work by treatment stages

	Harefield			Papworth		
	Transplant work			Transplant work		
	% of total	% of wte	£ p.a.	% of total	% of wte	£ p.a.
Assessment	59.0	7.7	943	39.4	20.1	2324
Operation to discharge	24.0	3.1	382	23.7	12.1	1398
Post discharge	17.0	2.2	273	36.8	18.7	2171
Totals	100.0	13.0	1598	100.0	50.8	5893

(catering, laundry and linen services) and non-patient related services (including administration, portering, cleaning, transport, estate management etc). In the short-run, the levels of service provided in the former category can be expected to be dependent upon patient numbers and hence are undoubtedly a relevant cost of the programme. In the absence of substantive information to the contrary we have treated these as if a transplant patient's day creates no greater or lesser demand on these services than the average patient day and have costed accordingly.

The so-called "non-patient related services" constitute a category of overheads that are rather less easily adjustable to patient levels. These overheads may well be irrelevant in the short-run, or for small changes in aggregate hospital workload, but do need to be included in a long-term planning context. Ideally we would apportion specific items within these overheads on the basis most relevant to the specific item: for example heating costs in relation to building volumes. But no such measures are appropriate to the nature of the transplant programmes as part of the overall surgical workloads. The apportionment of such overheads is inherently arbitrary. In the absence of any particular arguments to the contrary, we have also apportioned these in the standard way of a cost per inpatient day and per outpatient attendance.

5.15 Social work time

At both centres the hospital social worker is actively involved with patients in the programme. On our behalf the social workers associated with both programmes surveyed sample periods of their time, recording their involvement with transplant patients and related work. As TABLE 5.13 indicates, the distribution of transplant work by treatment stage is loaded towards the assessment period. Using this information on transplant work distribution and the overall wholetime-equivalent social worker involvement in the programme (which is rather different between the two centres) we have presented social work as an "overhead" to each programme, but divided by treatment stage.

5.16 "Transplant flats" in Harefield village

For some years two flats (and since January 1984 three flats) in the village of Harefield have been rented to provide accommodation for transplant patients who live far away, to permit earlier discharge whilst facilitating frequent outpatient contact (initially each weekday) with the hospital. No support services are provided in the flat except for cleaning. The total cost per annum for the flats for the year 1983–84 (including rent, rates, services, insurance and cleaning) was £4093. There was a 70 per cent occupancy during this period. This gives a cost of just £7.5 per night. This of course compares favourably with "hotel" costs within the hospital, or actual accommodation costs elsewhere. In addition, the flats provide conditions closer to those that the patient will experience on discharge home.

5.17 Capital costs: General

To provide an estimate of the additional cost attributable to use of capital, we have calculated a capital cost per day for a bed within a district general hospital necessarily based on national, and to some extent theoretical, data. It gives a figure relevant to the replacement cost of capital. The basis is the estimated capital costs of a "theoretical" *whole* hospital using DHSS building cost allowances for the various departments and allowing for on-costs of building, fees and equipment. (DHSS [1981]). The functional content of this theoretical hospital is based on an analysis of the departments found in the majority of a sample of 22 existing hospitals.

This exercise has been carried out for three sizes of hospital — 458 beds, 602 beds and 851 beds, and these produce a capital cost per bed (at a January 1984 price base) of £71 thousand, £61 thousand and £54 thousand per bed.

It is not practicable from this basis to attribute any of the capital costs to outpatients. These costs have then been discounted over a working life for the capital at 5 per cent (official discount rate) and adjusted to a cost per day reflecting an assumed 80 per cent occupancy. Following common conventions the buildings are assumed to have a sixty year life, the equipment fifteen. This gives a capital cost per bed-day of £13.8, £12.0 and £10.6 for the three sizes of hospital (458 beds, 602 beds, and 851 beds respectively).

This can be nothing more than an indicator, albeit one commonly used by the DHSS. A priori this calculation will give an underestimate for our purposes for the following reasons: (a) it takes no account of differential use of capital by different groups of patients within a partly acute hospital; (b) whilst it includes allowance for a suite of operating theatres (between 8–10) and all the related support services, these are not specifically geared to cardiac work. On the other hand it may overestimate the capital cost to the extent that for example recent evidence from particular nucleus hospital developments shows that in practice their capital costs can be significantly below the Departmental Cost Allowances embodied in these calculations. (DHSS [1984])

Nevertheless we would contend that a "balanced" hospital, even if theoretical, provides the best basis for assessing "typical" costs per bed, and we would take the middle of the three theoretical figures as the best available benchmark for capital cost, most likely to be relevant to broader strategic questions. However given its theoretical basis, we have chosen not to include this cost per day in any of the subsequent calculations, which can then be taken as simple revenue costs.

49

Table 5.14   Summary table of main unit costs: £   (1983–84 prices)

Item	Costing unit	Harefield	Papworth
		£	£
Surgical staff	Annual cost to the programme	37820	35360
Dental department	Annual cost to the programme	4450	—
Social Work staff	Annual cost to the programme	1600	5890
Transplant Outpatient nurse	Annual cost to the programme	7716	—
Consultant medical staff [Not included elsewhere]	Cost per worked hour	14.87	13.97
Nursing	Cost per day per patient by nursing dependency category	18.8- 221.9	18.0- 308.1
Ward/ITU consumables	As for nursing	10% of nursing cost	
Drugs/Pharmacy	Costs of specific drugs used	Purchase price including VAT plus dispensing overhead	
Cost of recipient operation [Including time of ALL staff involved except surgeons (above)]	Staff cost per operating hour	84.9	66.9
	Additional staff cost per op.	149.1	116.3
	Non-staff cost per operation	278.2	296.8
Respiratory Physiology	Cost per patient contact hour	22.1	22.1
Radiography etc [Incl. time of other staff involved]	Cost per standard workload unit, or per procedure as necessary	See Section 5.9	
Pathology etc	Cost per transplant request	See Table 5.10	
Electrocardiography [Incl. other stafff time]	Cost per procedure	See Table 5.11	
Blood products	Full cost per unit	See Table 5.12	
Physiotherapy	Cost per patient contact hour	5.7	7.8
General services Patient related	Cost per IP day/OP visit	4.32/ 0.42	5.73/ 1.21
Non patient related	Cost per IP day/OP visit	38.91/ 12.0	41.8/ 14.12
Transplant flats	Cost per occupied day	7.5	—
Capital	Theoretical cost per IP day	12.0	

5.18 Capital costs: Specific

As was noted in the previous Chapter, there is very little capital that can be argued to be specific to the transplant programme. Generally the programmes use the full range of resources normally available in a specialist cardiac centre, and little that is in any way peculiar to the transplant patients.

Perhaps the most apparent items are the "transplant rooms" adjacent to the two ITUs. In principle these are not exclusively for the use of transplant patients but in practice are rarely used by other patients. They provide an appropriate environment for the immediate postoperative period and incorporate clean air units. Conversion work for these cost approximately £50,000 at each centre.

A number of other items of building work and equipment have been charged to the programme at Harefield, including a gamma camera installation (£50,000); building work and equipment for a small immunology laboratory (approximately £25,000) and conversion of a room for transplant outpatients (£24,000). In addition other smaller items of equipment have been bought as a result of the increased cardiac workload, rather than as specific new require ments imposed by the programme.

These are simply indicative of some of the costs which have been incurred. We do not however feel it is appropriate to attempt to cost what future capital expenditure might be required at either centre, nor to estimate the capital costs that might be required if a new centre were to be set up. In each case, the functional requirements and the costs involved would be highly dependent on the level of spare capacity within the particular hospitals at the time. This spare capacity would depend on any other changes in workload.

5.19 Summary

In general we recorded in detail the resources used in the actual pattern of care and treatment provided for the specific patients being studied, and so attributed costs to individuals and by aggregation to the transplant programmes. Some items, which are specific to the programmes, but which we were unable to attribute to specific patients, have been treated as "programme overheads". Most importantly the time of the surgical teams devoted to the programmes has been estimated from detailed studies, and treated as an annual overhead; similarly the time of social work staff at the centres. General services costs have been apportioned in the usual manner.

The main units of costs for each centre are summarised in Table 5.14 and this provides a checklist against which to relate the actual cost estimates presented in the next Chapter.

In many cases, we know that the accuracy of the unit costs for some departments could be improved if more systematic data were available on the total workload and its distribution between patients. Sensitivity analysis, some of which is reported in Section 6.10, shows that further fine tuning of the estimates is unlikely to alter the overall picture, although it might significantly change particular elements of cost.

All our figures for the cost of staff reflect their total remuneration, including "out of hours" and "on call" supplements. But it is important to note that we have not been able to specifically adjust the unit costs for transplant patients to reflect any disproportionate level of "out of hours" or "on call" working they involve. This may lead to some underestimation of costs particularly in relation to the actual operation. The importance of this for the future depends on whether the programmes will continue to make greater call on "out of hours" staff time than is the case for other cardiac work.

Finally we would emphasise that it is not possible to put statistical confidence limits on our estimates of unit costs. The estimated totals quoted in subsequent Chapters, and, all the more so, their constituent elements, must be seen in the light of the detailed estimating procedures we have used.

6. Analysis of Costs by Treatment Stage and by Six-Month Periods Post Transplant

6.1 Introduction

We have adopted two approaches to costing the elements within the programmes. First we have estimated the costs of discrete patient episodes classified in terms of stages of treatment. Whilst conceptually this approach is quite straightforward, in practice some of the boundaries between stages are blurred, for example with the use of the "transplant flats" at Harefield. Nevertheless, we use this approach to estimate the costs of assessment, the costs between assessment and transplant, the period from transplant to discharge (including the costs of the recipient operation), and the donor operation.

Our second method is to use cross sectional data to build up profiles of the costs for patients in six month periods from transplantation. This approach enables us to report on the costs relating to a longer posttransplant experience than would be possible within the three years of this study by costing a cohort of patients from transplant.

Where a breakdown of costs is shown, we have categorised cost items using the same headings as in Chapter Five and including the items indicated there. We should reiterate that we have not included capital costs in any of the costings presented in this Report.

6.2 Costs by treatment stage: Assessment

The cost calculations for the assessment stage are summarised in TABLE 6.1 and use the costing conventions outlined in Chapter Five. The costs presented in this table are based on data for 65 assessments at Harefield, and 49 at Papworth during the period 1st July 1983 — 30th June 1984. Within these data sets all observations are patient specific including the levels of nursing dependency. The figures show that during this period the average cost of an assessment has been £1180 at Harefield and £429 at Papworth.

It must be remembered that these figures do not include the cost of the time of the transplant surgeons involved in the assessment, nor of social work, both of which have been treated as overheads to the programme. Nor do they necessarily reflect the differences in overall costs to the NHS (see Chapter Seven).

During the periods used for this costing, the average length of assessment at Papworth was 3.6 days and at Harefield 9.7 days. Thus the differences in costs between the centres reflect closely the proportionate differences in length of stay.

Earlier costing, carried out on a smaller sample of patients from the previous eighteen months with less well-developed data sources, suggests that the costs at assessment at Harefield have fallen significantly whilst those at Papworth have remained fairly constant in real terms, and possibly risen slightly. Again such observations on cost relativities are in line with the firm data on differences in length of stay.

Table 6.1: Average costs per patient: Assessment (1 July 1983 – 30 June 1984)

(1983 – 84 prices)

	Assessment	
	Harefield (N = 65)	Papworth (N = 49)
	£	£
Nursing	390	83
Consumables	39	8
Drugs	33	7
Respiratory physiology	25	2
Radiography etc	64	12
Pathology etc	181	120
Electrocardiography	20	1
Other	11	27
Sub-total	762	260
General services	418	169
Grand total	1180	429

6.3 Costs by treatment stage: Period between assessment and transplant

Patients at this stage in the programme, accounted for 34 bed days at Papworth in the 31 months up to September 1984. Of these, only three days were in 1984 and we have not attempted to cost them.

In the early stages of the programme it was common for patients to "wait" as inpatients in Harefield rather than return to their local referring hospital, and whilst the propensity to keep patients at Harefield has declined, in 1984 a total of some 134 inpatient days were spent "waiting" there.

TABLE 6.2 presents the average costs for 17 patients, who were too ill to be at home, and who spent a period between assessment and transplant in Harefield during the year July 1983 – June 1984. The length of this "waiting" stay varied between two and 41 days. The average was 12 days. The cost breakdown reflects that there is relatively little treatment activity or testing involved; the costs are mainly for fairly high dependency nursing.

It should also be stressed that this cost per patient is averaged only over those who spent some time waiting. If it were calculated on the basis of the total number of patients at that stage in the programme, the average costs per patient presented in TABLE 6.2 would need to be divided by a factor of six to seven.

6.4 Costs by treatment stage: Transplant to discharge home

TABLE 6.3 presents the costs for transplant to discharge, consisting of one column of figures for Papworth but two for Harefield, for which the second represents the average period of stay in the "transplant flats". The costs are based on 47 transplant patients at Harefield and 21 at Papworth who were all discharged alive. As for the assessment costs, the figures are based on patient specific recording of resource usage. The costs for the transplant flats are averaged over that total of 47 transplant patients, although only 38 spent a period in the flats. This means that the two totals for Harefield can be added and com-

Table 6.2: Average cost per patient: "Waiting" (1 July 1983–30 June 1984)

(1983–84 prices)

	"Waiting"
	Harefield (N = 17)
	£
Nursing	882
Consumables	88
Drugs	69
Respiratory physiology	0
Radiography etc	31
Pathology	42
Electrocardiography	7
Sub-total	1119
General services	519
Grand total	1638

pared (to the extent that any such comparison is valid) with the Papworth figures. Making this comparison, the cost totals are £6,181 for Harefield and £11,158 for Papworth.

These totals again reflect significant differences in the length of stay. For these costed groups of patients (all patients between July 1983 and June 1984) we are comparing a stay in hospital of 14.2 days at Harefield with a stay of 44.2 days at Papworth. It is interesting to note how consistently the differences in cost occur in almost all items. The considerably higher cost of the recipient operation for Papworth is explained almost entirely by the cost of the pacemaker which is routinely inserted with the transplanted heart at Papworth, a practice not followed at Harefield. The costs are low for the period in the flats at Harefield (for patients who would not otherwise be able to make daily outpatient visits in the first week or so). No nursing or other support is provided in the flats; the costs shown are for drugs, tests carried out at outpatient visits and the general services cost of those outpatient visits and the cost per day of the flats.

Again we have compared these figures with estimates we made earlier for the same transplant stage based on observations in the period January 1982–June 1983. Whilst accurate comparison of costs between the two periods is not possible, because we did not have full data collection systems (for example for ITU nursing dependency) in place during the earlier period, it is clear that (in keeping with the trends we have identified) the costs at Harefield have fallen considerably, whilst those at Papworth have remained of the same order.

6.5 Costs by treatment stage: Transplant operation to death

All the data in the previous section related to patients discharged alive. We have separately analysed the costs of those who died in hospital (TABLE 6.4). These figures are based on just four cases at Harefield and three at Papworth in the year

54

Table 6.3   Average costs per patient: Operation to discharge (1 July 1983 – 30 June 1984)

(1983 – 84 Prices)

	Transplant operation to discharge		
	Harefield (N = 47)		Papworth (N = 21)
	Hospital £	Flats £	£
Nursing	1490	—	2735
Consumables	149	—	273
Drugs	767	452	1445
Recipient Operation	934	—	1711
Respiratory Physiology	47	—	—
Radiography etc	170	68	584
Pathology etc	642	153	1656
Blood Products	377	—	465
Electrocardiography	66	17	76
Physiotherapy	26	—	110
Sub-Total	4668	691	9055
General Services	615	207	2103
Grand Total	5283	898	11158

to June 1984, so the figures whilst accurate may be unrepresentative for the future. They should be seen as little more than indicative of the fact that the cost of patients who die in hospital may be quite different from that of patients discharged alive.

6.6 Costs by treatment stage: Donor operation

Our cost figures for transplant to discharge include the costs of the recipient operation, but exclude those of the donor operation.

There are three main costs to the transplantation centres:

(i) the time of the team who go to remove the donor heart;

(ii) the time of support staff involved in co-ordinating the operation and liaising with the donor hospital, and the other parties involved;

(iii) the costs of travel (if charged to the transplantation centre).

Other costs incurred by the donor's hospital will be separately considered in Chapter Seven.

Normally the team that goes to the donor hospital consists of a consultant surgeon and a senior technician who also acts as co-ordinator. In addition the Papworth team includes a junior surgeon and a nurse, whereas the Harefield team tends to make greater use of donor hospital personnel.

The time of the surgeons has been treated as an overhead so should not be separately attributed to the donor operation. On average the time between departure from and arrival back at the centre is 4.3 hours at Harefield and 5.0 hours at Papworth and the costs of this time for the teams (other than the surgeons) is therefore estimated at £39 (Harefield) and £70 (Papworth).

The time spent in co-ordination is estimated to be on average 11.2 hours per donor operation. This gives a time cost of £102, based on a senior technician's salary, but appreciating that the co-ordination may in practice be done by one of

Table 6.4   Average costs per patient: Operation to death (1 July 1983–30 June 1984)

(1983–84 prices)

	Transplant operation to death	
	Harefield (N = 4)	Papworth (N = 3)
	£	£
Nursing	4056	2226
Consumables	406	223
Drugs	1021	928
Recipient operation	984	1814
Respiratory physiology	178	—
Radiography etc	414	390
Pathology etc	1118	1106
Blood products	924	849
Electrocardiography	98	15
Physiotherapy	50	34
Sub-total	9249	7584
General services	821	602
Grand total	10071	8187

a number of different staff.

The large degree of variability in the distances to donor hospitals, and the means of transporting both the donor teams and donor hearts, mitigates against the reporting of a simple average travel cost. However, the available data suggests that average travel costs per donor operation lie between £300 to £600. This reflects the fact that on a number of occasions a commercial service is used whilst in the remainder some non-commercial service — often the St. John Ambulance Service Air Wing or the police — provide travel facilities.

Together the estimates for these three main elements, plus the additional cost of donor tissue typing, suggest a cost of around £490 to £800 per donor operation falling on the transplant centres.

6.7 The concept of cross-sectional views

Costing by treatment stage, we are able to produce fairly satisfactory figures for assessment and for the immediate postoperative inpatient care, and to give indicative figures for the waiting period and for the donor operation. However it is important to build up a picture of the likely long-term costs of transplant patients, using the limited evidence that is available from the existing "long-term" survivors.

Within the period of our prospective resource use data collection, (ie from January 1st 1982 up to a cut-off point of 30th June 1984) we have had, so to speak, a 30 month "window" onto a continuing programme enabling us to observe patients at different posttransplant periods. By grouping observations of those patients in terms of standard six-month periods from the date of each patient's transplant, we are able to build up a composite picture of posttransplant costs. These reflect our observations of patients who have been transplanted at different stages in the programme, and we can split these observations into four sequential "cross-sectional" views of the cost profiles for posttransplant patients.

This "quasi cross-sectional" approach gives the best substitute for a longitudinal view of a cohort of patients over their whole posttransplant survival period, the latter being an approach that was not feasible within the three year limit to the whole study.

6.8 The pattern and numbers of the observations

This "quasi cross-sectional" approach is illustrated in TABLE 6.5. Thus for example, for any patients transplanted in the first half of 1981 we would not have cost data for the first postoperative year but we would have observations for four periods of six months posttransplant namely 13–18 months, 19–24 months, 25–30 months, and 31–36 months. These would contribute to the "cross-sectional views" I, II, III and IV respectively. It will be noted that only patients transplanted up to the end of December 1983, are included in this analysis.

The maximum size of any of these groups is determined by the number of transplants performed in the relevant six-months period. The actual size depends upon the length of survival of the particular patients. TABLE 6.6 gives the numbers in each group who are alive for the whole six-month period. Inevitably the numbers in each cell are small, but the data from each of the four sequential

Table 6.5   The basis of the cross section views:
The identification of which groups of patients contribute observations to each cross section view based on their date of transplantation.

	Six-month posttransplant periods ·								
	TX−6	7−12	13−18	19−24	25−30	31−36	37−42	43−48	49−54
Cross Section View I	1982/I	1981/II	1981/I	1980/II	1980/I	1979/II	—	—	—
Cross Section View II	1982/II	1982/I	1981/II	1981/I	1980/II	1980/I	1979/II	—	—
Cross Section View III	1983/I	1982/II	1982/I	1981/II	1981/I	1980/II	1980/I	1979/II	—
Cross Section View IV	1983/II	1983/I	1982/II	1982/I	1981/II	1981/I	1980/II	1980/I	1979/II

Table 6.6   Number of cost observations (Patients) by six-month periods posttransplant: Patients alive throughout six-month period

	Six-month Posttransplant Periods								
	TX−6	7−12	13−18	19−24	25−30	31−36	37−42	43−48	49−54
Harefield:									
Cross Section View I	8	5	—	2	1	—	—	—	—
Cross Section View II	4	8	4	—	2	1	—	—	—
Cross Section View III	15	4	8	3	—	2	1	—	—
Cross Section View IV	12	15	4	8	3	—	2	1	—
Total	39	32	16	13	6	3	3	1	—
Papworth:									
Cross Section View I	7	1	5	2	3	1	—	—	—
Cross Section View II	4	7	1	5	2	3	1	—	— ·
Cross Section View III	8	3	7	1	5	2	2	1	—
Cross Section View IV	7	8	3	7	1	5	2	2	1
Total	26	20	16	15	11	11	5	3	1

Table 6.7: Number of cost observations (patients) by six-month periods posttransplant: Deaths during six-month period

	TX−6	7−12	13−18	19−24	25−30	31−36	37−42	43−48	49−54

	TX−6	7−12	13−18	19−24	25−30	31−36	37−42	43−48	49−54
Harefield:	15	-	1	1	-	-	-	-	-
Papworth:	8	1	2	-	-	1	1	-	-

Six-month Posttransplant Periods

"views" can be amalgamated to increase the sample base (but recognising that this then obscures any change in the cost profile as the programme and patterns of treatment have developed).

In addition we have cost data for six-month periods in which patients died. These very few observations are also presented by the six-month period posttransplant in which the patient died, but they have not been disaggregated by "cross section view" (TABLE 6.7).

6.9 The cost analysis by six month periods after transplantation

The results of this cost analysis are summarised in TABLE 6.8. The figures include all the costs associated with their inpatient stays at, and outpatient visits to, the transplant centres, subject only to the exclusion of the same costs as in the previous sections — overheads to the programme and capital. In addition patient specific estimates of the full drug costs of the patients are included irrespective of from where the drugs were dispensed. However the costs of outpatient visits to other hospitals are not included, but are discussed specifically in Chapter Seven. The TABLE shows that for Harefield patients the average cost for the first six months (including the cost of the transplant operation itself and the immediate inpatient care) has been £12.4 thousand per patient whilst the equivalent average figure for Papworth has been £15.0 thousand. The average cost of subsequent six month periods at Harefield appears to decline from £2.7 thousand for 7−12 months, to £1.1 thousand for the period 25−30 months. Similarly for Papworth the cost figures fall from £2.9 thousand to £1.2 thousand. For periods after 25−30 months at Harefield and 31−36 months at Papworth the figures are based on so few observations that they must be treated with extreme caution. In looking to the future the change over time is interesting and relevant. Each cross-section view presents a more recent picture. At Harefield, but to a lesser extent Papworth, there has been a significant decline in the costs of the first six month period. However at both centres the subsequent costs have been rising, mainly reflecting the costs associated with the use of Cyclosporin A.

A breakdown of the cost totals is presented in TABLE 6.9 for cross section view IV which gives the most recent picture.

All the preceding cost figures are for patients who survived the whole of the relevant six month periods. We have separately analysed costs for patients who have died during the particular six month period; these are summarised in TABLE 6.10. It is extremely difficult to generalise from these except perhaps to make two points:

(a) because the majority of patients who die in the first six month period (TX−6) do so as inpatients it is reasonable to compare this six month period with

Table 6.8: **Average costs per patient by six-month periods posttransplant**

£ thousands

	Six-month posttransplant periods								
	TX–6	7–12	13–18	19–24	25–30	31–36	37–42	43–48	49–54
Harefield:									
Cross Section View I	16.15	2.50	—	0.84	1.01	—	—	—	—
Cross Section View II	13.10	2.24	1.17	—	1.55	0.92	—	—	—
Cross Section View III	11.75	2.87	2.42	1.49	—	1.51	1.45	—	—
Cross Section View IV	10.37	3.04	2.80	1.80	0.76	—	0.23	1.17	—
Weighted Average	12.37	2.73	2.20	1.58	1.07	1.31	0.64	1.17	—
Papworth:									
Cross Section View I	16.42	1.10	0.88	0.66	0.87	0.58	—	—	—
Cross Section View II	13.99	3.37	1.02	0.51	0.81	1.35	0.94	—	—
Cross Section View III	14.65	2.85	2.08	0.48	1.50	0.52	1.01	7.28	—
Cross Section View IV	14.42	2.76	1.98	1.99	1.39	1.08	1.03	0.53	2.75
Weighted Average	14.96	2.91	1.62	1.22	1.19	1.01	1.00	2.78	2.75

TABLE 6.4 which presents costs for all patients who died prior to discharge;

(b) for deaths in later periods there is immense variability depending on the date of death within the fixed six month period, and whether the death occurred suddenly at home or after a lengthy period of treatment in hospital for rejection or infection.

6.10 Sensitivity analyses

It is evident from the detail in Chapter Five that our unit costs involve a number of assumptions and estimates. In some cases valid alternative conventions are available and could have been used. We do not think it helpful to pursue each of these and proffer a whole series of alternative estimates. Instead we have generally preferred to use our professional judgement and to adopt what seems to us to be the most appropriate unit cost estimates.

Nevertheless for illustrative purposes we have analysed the sensitivity of our main results for the costs of assessment, and of operation to discharge, to certain alternative assumptions about unit costs. These analyses are presented in TABLE 6.11.

Initially we focussed on nursing costs as one of the largest cost items. The first test of sensitivity [(A) FIGURE 6.11] was the effect of excluding the cost of pupil and student nurses, on the basis of the argument that they were undergoing training rather than contributing directly to the nursing service. The effect of this change on the total costs of assessment and of transplant to discharge is a small reduction, but in all cases the percentage change is less than 3 per cent.

The second test of sensitivity we report (B) looked at the effect of applying the simple average nursing cost per inpatient day for each hospital rather than the costs reflecting the observed weighting related to nursing dependency. The effect of this is, not surprisingly, more dramatic. For assessment patients at Harefield the effect is a slight reduction in cost implying that assessment patients are slightly more "nursing dependent" than the average for the hospital. The difference is even greater for the Papworth transplant to discharge and most

Table 6.9: Average costs per patient by six-month periods posttransplant: Cross section view IV

£

	TX-6	7-12	13-18	19-24	25-30	31-36	37-42	43-48	49-54
Harefield:									
Nursing	1914	143	87	53	52	—	51	102	—
Consumables	191	14	9	5	5	—	5	10	—
Drugs	3768	1969	2214	1338	376	—	639	668	—
Recipient Operation	976	51*	—	—	—	—	—	—	—
Respiratory Physio.	52	1	—	—	—	—	—	—	—
Radiography etc	539	214	121	70	78	—	59	118	—
Pathology etc	1216	253	177	128	79	—	36	72	—
Blood Products	376	10	—	—	—	—	—	—	—
Electrocardiography	134	80	55	45	44	—	17	69	—
Physiotherapy	25	1	—	—	—	—	—	—	—
Sub-total	9191	2737	2663	1640	635	—	801	1039	—
General services	1181	306	138	162	124	—	65	130	—
Grand total	10372	3043	2801	1802	759	—	866	1168	—
Papworth:									
Nursing	3205	106	17	73	210	141	50	—	286
Consumables	320	11	2	7	21	14	5	—	29
Drugs	2815	2121	1768	1515	438	361	505	495	529
Recipient operation	1691	—	—	—	—	—	—	—	—
Respiratory physio.	—	—	—	—	—	—	—	—	—
Radiography etc	822	124	87	27	264	114	259	3	546
Pathology etc	2237	177	44	188	102	126	85	9	338
Blood products	601	—	—	—	—	—	—	—	—
Electrocardiography	100	8	2	6	5	9	2	4	26
Physiotherapy	138	—	—	—	—	—	—	—	—
Sub-total	11928	2546	1919	1816	1040	765	905	511	1753
General services	2497	217	64	172	348	311	126	23	1001
Grand total	14425	2763	1983	1988	1388	1076	1031	534	2754

* One patient in group was operated on to remove heterotopic transplant

Table 6.10 Average costs per patient by six-month periods posttransplant: deaths during six-months period

£ thousands

	TX-6	7-12	13-18	19-24	25-30	31-36	37-42	43-48	49-54
Harefield:	11.12	—	15.07	0.51	—	—	—	—	—
Papworth:	12.01	6.81	1.00	—	—	1.17	10.06	—	—

marked for Harefield transplant to discharge. A simple average nursing cost would reduce the latter estimate by 20 per cent. This reflects the high average level of nursing during this relative short postoperative inpatient stay. These calculations do not in any way lead us to doubt the validity of our approach and the appropriateness of our figures, but they do emphasise the impact that such differentiation of nursing dependency has on cost estimates. It is important to re-

Table 6.11: Sensitivity analyses of total costs for assessment and for transplant to discharge

	Assessment		Transplant to discharge	
	Harefield	Papworth	Harefield	Papworth
Total Cost (Baseline)	£1180	£429	£5283	£11158
A. Exclusion of costs of				
Pupil/Student nurses	£1157	£428	£5138	£11036
% Change in total costs	− 1.9	− 0.3	− 2.7	− 1.1
B. Use of Hospital average				
cost per nursing day	£1143	£493	£4220	£10089
% Change in total costs	− 3.1	+ 14.9	− 20.1	− 9.6
C. "Exchange of unit costs"	£1036	£520	£4765	£13220
% Change in total costs	− 12.2	+ 21.2	− 9.8	+ 18.5

member this particularly if comparisons are made with other estimates that are not so appropriately adjusted.

Finally, we wanted to confirm that the differences in costs between the centres are a product of the differences in resources used rather than differences in the unit costs at the two centres. Therefore in the third reported analysis (C), we applied the Harefield unit costs to the Papworth resource usage data and vice-versa. This produces some interesting differences. Not surprisingly, given such factors as London Allowances on pay etc, the Papworth unit costs decrease the Harefield totals and the Harefield unit costs increase the totals for Papworth. The extent of the change, however, is rather greater than could be easily explained by that factor alone. The sensitivity analysis emphasise the important fact that there are substantive differences between the centres in the resources used at assessment and in the period from transplant to discharge.

6.11 Summary

Costs have been presented in two forms, first in terms of discrete patient episodes classified by stage of treatment, and second in cross sectional views of patient experience, classified in six-month periods from the operation.

Estimates of the costs incurred at assessment were based on those patients assessed during the period July 1983 – June 1984: 65 at Harefield and 49 at Papworth. Excluding the "programme overheads", most particularly the time of the surgeons and the social worker, the average costs were £1,180 at Harefield and £429 at Papworth respectively, reflecting the very different lengths of inpatient stay as reported in Chapter Three. In addition, a small number of patients, who were too ill to wait at home, spent periods between assessment and transplant in Harefield. For 17 such patients (during the period July 1983 – June 1984) the average cost was estimated at £1,638.

The estimated costs per patient for the period from transplant to discharge alive, averaged £5,283 (over 14.2 days) at Harefield and £11,158 (over 44.2 days) at Papworth (based on 47 and 21 patients respectively, again from the year July 1983 – June 1984). In addition at Harefield, the average cost per patient of the stay in the "transplant flats" was £898, giving a total estimate of £6,181 from transplant to discharge home.

The overall cost to the transplant centre relating to the donor operation is between £490 and £800, mainly related to travel and therefore very variable depending upon distance and mode of transport. (Again, as with all these figures, the time of the surgeons is not included).

Using the cross sectional approach of analysing costs by six-month periods after operation, for the most recent group of patients that we costed the average cost of the first six months after transplant has been £10.4 thousand at Harefield and £14.4 thousand at Papworth (including the costs of all drugs wherever dispensed, and all IP or OP visits to the transplant centres but *not* to any local hospitals). For the second six months, the figures are £3.0 and £2.8 thousand respectively. Subsequent periods show a declining cost but may be less representative of the long-term costs of patients because they are based on the experience of patients transplanted earlier in the programme and who generally have not been receiving the expensive immunosuppressive drug, Cyclosporin A. The long term costs of treatment for recent patients receiving this drug will be considerably higher and probably closer to our figures for the second six months.

Sensitivity analysis suggests that the general orders of magnitude and the major differences would not be significantly changed by adopting alternative detailed assumptions in the costings. It confirms that the estimated differences in costs reflect real differences in the volume of resources used per patient at the two centres both at assessment and post transplant, and that they are not simply a product of differences in unit costs.

7. 'Net' Costs to the NHS and Costs Elsewhere in the Public Sector

7.1 Introduction

The cost tables presented in Chapter Six are principally concerned with costs incurred at the Centres, although certain items of cost, it was noted, do not normally fall on the hospitals' budgets. However, in addition, the tables note a number of items of health service expenditure that are incurred away from the Centres. For example, the tables presenting costs by six month periods posttransplant include the costs of posttransplant drugs no matter where they are dispensed.

This Chapter cautiously explores the likely extent of such additional costs elsewhere and the extent to which certain costs, that would anyway have been incurred, should be netted off quoted figures in assessing the net cost to the NHS. Figures on costs to be added to or netted off those presented in Chapter Six have to be extremely tentative in that we have no control group against which unequivocally to compare the costs of the transplant patients. They have to be based on judgements of what would otherwise have been the treatment/management pattern for those patients. Finally, we consider briefly any major costs falling on the rest of the public sector.

7.2 Costs prior to referral

Essentially, we take the significant costs of the programme as commencing at assessment. However we carried out a survey of a sample of 58 consultants who had referred patients to the programmes during 1983 (and whose patients had been assessed) to establish whether or not additional procedures, tests or time had been incurred with respect to potential transplant patients at various stages that would not otherwise have been carried out on those patients. The results are summarised in TABLE 7.1.

Prior to *referral* approximately one quarter of the respondents who had referred patients to Harefield indicated that some additional procedure had been carried out. For Papworth one half of the respondents indicated some additional procedure, consultation or interviews, but for half of these it was only additional discussions with patients and family which took place. The diagnostic procedures most frequently mentioned were right heart catheterisation, angiography, and measurement of pulmonary vascular resistance. It is clear that some additional resources are employed at this stage, but in terms of additional cost to the "routine" management of these cardiac patients the increases would appear to be marginal. Costs prior to referral can probably be ignored.

7.3 Costs between referral and assessment

At this stage, one quarter of each centre's respondents indicated that some additional tests or monitoring had been carried out. Usually, but not always, this was as a result of a specific request from the transplantation centre. A variety of specific tests or procedures were cited but again, in terms of a cost per patient assessed, the figures would be low. Potentially such costs may become more important however in that they will be affected by the policies of the transplant centres.

Table 7.1:   Survey of referring doctors

Question 1:

Prior to referral of the patient(s) to one of the Transplant Surgeons, did you do anything additional (or different) in relation to that patient because you were planning to refer him to be considered for a heart transplant? If so, please indicate the nature of the additional tests, procedures, interviews or whatever.

Question 2A:

Following referral but prior to the patient's formal assessment at Harefield or Papworth did you do anything additional (or different) because the patient had been accepted for assessment for transplant?

Question 2B:

If so, was any of the above as a result of a specific request from the Transplant Centre?

Question 3:

If your patient(s) was accepted for transplant, did the acceptance (definite or provisional) affect your managment of the patient in the period between formal assessment at the Transplant Centre and the eventual transplant operation (or death if that occurred before a transplant operation could take place)?

	Harefield		Papworth	
Number Surveyed:	26		32	
Number of responses:	17		26	
Response rate:	65%		81%	
Responses:	NO.	%	NO.	%
'No' to all three questions	9	52.9	6	23.1
'Yes' to one or more questions	8	47.1	20	76.9
Questions: 1	4		14	
2A	4		7	
2B	3		6	
3	2		7	

7.4 Costs between acceptance and tranplant

At this stage 12 per cent of Harefield respondents and 27 per cent of Papworth respondents indicated that their management of the patient had been affected by his/her acceptance for transplant, but this seemed mainly to be a question of closer monitoring (extra outpatient visits), and additional interviews or discussions involving principally the social worker. Perhaps most significantly from a cost point of view there was a suggestion that patients may have spent somewhat longer as inpatients at the referring hospital at this stage than would otherwise have been the case. Given the inevitably hypothetical nature of our question and of the answers to it, it is inappropriate to attempt to provide a specific estimate but it seems likely that small but significant additional costs may typically be incurred at this stage.

Additionally and quite separately we have estimated the health service resources consumed on average during the period after assessment by patients definitely accepted for transplant. These figures are based on sample two-week "diaries" completed for us every three months post assessment by the patients. The results are summarised in TABLE 7.2. Although the samples are rather small a reasonable picture emerges. The results suggest a fairly high call on health service resources for accepted patients: expressed as weekly rates, drug costs of around £10/£12; approximately fortnightly to monthly visits to an outpatient clinic, from a GP, and a further visit to a GP once a month; a visit once every month or two months by a social worker or nurse, and an average of just over one day a month in another hospital for Papworth patients, but less frequently for Harefield patients. Whilst there are reasons to believe that these latter figures may be underestimates as a result of bias in the sample towards those who were "well" at home, the differences tally with the picture of a greater propensity to admit patients to Harefield itself, during this period beween transplant and assessment. (Cost figures for these stays were given in TABLE 6.2.) In the absence of a "medically managed" control group these figures for patients who have been assessed and accepted, but not yet transplanted, also have to serve as an indication of what the pattern of resource usage might be for transplant patients without surgery.

Table 7.2 Resources used by patients after assessment: Average per two week sample period for definitely accepted patients.

	Harefield (N = 29)	Papworth (N = 48)
Cost of Drugs	£19.19	£23.66
Numbers of:		
— Outpatient visits	0.6	0.9
— Visits to GP	0.4	0.5
— Home visits by GP	0.4	1.0
— Other contacts with nurse, community social worker, health visitor	0.2	0.4
— Inpatient days at other hospitals	0.2	0.6

7.5 Cost to the donor's hospital of the donor operation

The donor operation involes the donor centre in two main elements of cost. The first relates to the period from the brain death of the donor to the beginning of the operation and the second to the operation itself. We estimate the average time from brain death to donor operation to have been 9.2 hours, and during this time period typically the donor is under the care of an ITU nurse. (We have costed this at the average of the Harefield and Papworth nursing costs for a patient in ITU care group A.) In addition, a junior hospital doctor or transplant co-ordinator is normally involved throughout the period in co-ordinating with the transplant teams and a consultant is likely to be involved for half the time. This gives an average cost of £220.

A sample of donor operations including the time taken to remove other organs lasted on average two hours and this represents a cost of approximately £65 for the basic staff from the donor hospital who are needed in theatre: an anaesthetist, 2/3 nurses and two operation department assistants.

This gives an identifiable cost of around £285 per donor operation to the donor hospital. However it must be stressed that in 97 per cent of cases the kidneys are also removed and these costs need to be seen as relating to the procurement of all the organs removed. The marginal cost of excising the heart would just be any extra time involved in co-ordinating (or delay to the operation) as a result of the desire to remove the heart, and the extra time added of the surgery which is estimated at about twenty-five minutes.

In addition to the costs at the donor hospital some costs are also incurred by UK Transplant Service (see Section 2.2).

7.6 Posttransplant

The TABLES 6.8 to 6.10 presenting the cross section analysis by six month group include two elements of drug costs: those provided in hospital during inpatient periods, and drug costs in the community. The latter again use estimates based on two week sample periods recorded for us in diaries. These figures emphasise the long term costs of the Cyclosporin A based drug therapy which now appears to average at least £1,500 per patient per six-month period.

In addition, we have estimates of the number of outpatient visits made to local hospitals. The estimate for Harefield is again based on two week sample periods; for Papworth the figures are based on detailed guidelines prepared by the surgeons and provided to transplant patients' local doctors, which clearly set out a pattern of *routine* local outpatient visits to dovetail with the visits to Papworth. For comparison TABLE 7.3 shows the average numbers of outpatient visits reflected in the costing by six-month periods in the preceeding chapter, and also the number of additional OP visits to other hospitals, which were not included in our basic costs. These show much lower rates for Papworth patients than for Harefield in terms of outpatient visits both to the transplant centre and to their local hospitals. The "theoretical routine" rate for Papworth may of course underestimate the number of visits actually made. To give an indicative estimate of the costs of these, the national average cost per outpatient visit, on a comparable price basis is around £20.00 (DHSS [1984b]). When this unit cost is applied it appears that an additional cost per six-month period for Papworth patients is £90.00 in the period 7–12 months reducing to a longer term figure of around £50.00 relating to outpatient visits elsewhere. On the Harefield data, the first six months are the most expensive in terms of these additional outpatient visits with costs amounting to some £460; this figure reduces to an estimated £270 in the period 7–12 months, and further declines subsequently to about £120 per six-month period.

7.7 Other public sector costs

From the outset we agreed to limit our study by not attempting to measure the broader public sector effects of the programme. In particular we have not collected data on the financial circumstances of patients and the different calls on social security benefits. In a strict sense such benefits are transfer payments from one group (tax-payers) to another (beneficiaries) and as such do not represent a net call on resources. For this reason it would have been inappropriate in a study of resource costs to focus on social security issues. In practical terms, the matter may be of policy interest but its study would require very detailed collection of personal data from the families of patients on their incomes, benefits, savings etc and might have jeopardised the very high level of co-operation we received from the patients on other more central issues.

Three aspects of public sector costs however merit attention at this point although we do not have adequate data to cost them.

Table 7.3.   Number of outpatient visits by six-month periods posttransplant

	TX-6	7-12	13-18	19-24	25-30	31-36	37-42	43-48	49-54
Harefield patients:									
Visits to Harefield									
Cross section view I	29.0	28.2	—	0.5	0.0	—	—	—	—
Cross section view II	23.3	6.8	13.5	—	0.0	1.0	—	—	—
Cross section view III	9.5	5.0	7.6	5.0	—	0.5	0.0	—	—
Cross section view IV	17.4	7.5	3.3	7.4	3.0	—	N/D	0.0	—
Visits to local hospital									
Cross section view I	13.3	3.3	—	5.0	13.0	—	—	—	—
Cross section view II	17.5	19.3	4.3	—	13.0	8.0	—	—	—
Cross section view III	17.9	19.5	10.7	6.3	—	19.0	6.0	—	—
Cross section view IV	23.2	13.4	9.8	9.2	6.5	—	N/D	6.0	—
Papworth patients:									
Visits to Papworth									
Cross section view I	4.0	4.0	2.0	3.0	1.7	3.0	—	—	—
Cross section view II	6.0	3.9	1.6	2.8	1.0	1.7	1.0	—	—
Cross section view III	5.5	2.8	2.1	1.0	1.4	2.5	1.5	4.0	—
Cross section view IV	6.6	3.0	2.0	1.9	1.0	2.5	2.0	1.5	25.0
Visits to local hospital									
"Routine pattern"	3.0	4.3	3.0	3.0	2.2	2.2	2.2	2.2	2.2

A. *Ambulance/Transport costs*

We have specifically referred only to the travel costs of the team that goes to obtain the donor heart. However, given the geographical dispersion of patients shown in Chapter Two, it is obvious that the programme involves them in considerable travel for assessment, for the operation itself, and for subsequent inpatient and outpatient visits. The travel arrangements vary depending amongst other things upon the state of health of the patient at the time and the alternative transport available for the particular journey. Considerable use is made of ambulances, but also private cars and public transport. The costs tend to be very dispersed amongst different authorities and the individuals concerned, and we feel unable to make a satisfactory estimate.

B. *Police escorts*

Even in costing the travel associated with the donor operation we were unable to include the costs of police escorts or for police transport where this has been used. This tends to be for the shorter journeys — particularly from London hospitals or from an airport.

C. *Social work costs*

We set out in Chapter Five the costs associated with the hospital social workers, and suggested that their time might best be seen as an overhead [TABLE 5.13].

(These costs are met by the local authorities rather than the Health Authorities). In addition there are costs of social work support for the patient at home or at his local hospital. In that psychosocial stability is a criterion for the selection of a patient for transplantation, and given the obvious strain the disease and the prospect of the procedure can place on families, local social work support is an integral part of the programme and needs to be planned for.

7.8 Summary

In the absence of a control group against which to unequivocally compare the costs of care provided to heart transplant patients, we do not feel able to provide firm estimates of the costs that should be netted off the figures quoted in the previous chapter, or should be added to allow for care provided elsewhere, that would not otherwise have been provided to patients who are involved in the transplant programmes. However on the basis of the professional judgement of a sample of referring consultants, and on information from patient diaries and interviews we have attempted to indicate the sorts of resources involved.

We have noted what extra resources appear to have been employed at the hospitals of patients referred for possible transplant prior to their referral, during the period from referral to assessment, and from assessment to transplant. Whilst there is evidence that some extra investigations and tests were carried out, some of them at the request of the transplant centres, the net impact on the overall costs of transplantation is probably marginal.

We have also looked at the costs to the donor's hospital of the donor operation. We have estimated an identifiable cost of around £285 per donor operation. However this should properly be seen as a joint cost for the procurement of all the organs removed. [In 97 per cent of cases the kidneys were also removed.]

The figures presented in Chapter Six for costs per six-month period posttransplant already include the costs of all drugs wherever dispensed. To these costs however should be added the cost of outpatient visits to local hospitals. We have estimated the number of these for Harefield and for Papworth patients using rather different methods. Applying a national average cost per OP visit of approximately £20.00, these visits involve an additional cost for Harefield patients of approximately £460 in the first six months after transplant reducing over time to about £120 per six month period. For Papworth patients the "routine pattern" of visits to local hospitals adds to the costs a maximum of about £90 in the period 7–12 months, reducing to around £50 subsequently.

8. Patient Survival

[N.B. Uniquely this Chapter is followed by a series of detailed technical notes referenced in the text by a number in square brackets.]

8.1 Introduction

Cardiac transplantation is seen as offering 'a new lease of life' to very ill patients for whom the prognosis without transplantation would be very poor; this concept includes two aspects of benefit — duration and quality of life. This Chapter deals with duration in terms of analyses of survival.

In the first part we present data on post-transplant survival for each programme, and for the two combined in terms of individual survival and cumulative survival curves. We compare the survival probabilities of the two programmes, and of the combined data with that of the Stanford Heart Transplant Programme. We then attempt to compare the survival experience of different "groups" of transplanted patients; in particular, patients are grouped by transplant chronology to determine whether survival is improving over time. Finally we use multi-variate analysis to identify other relevant co-variates (or "risk factors") such as age of recipient and/or donor, that may influence patient survival.

In the final section we focus on the fundamental question of the extent to which transplantation increases survival. We summarise the attempts that have been made, in the context of the early data from the Stanford Program, to test the hypothesis statistically, given that no randomised control group exists to provide a direct comparison. We then apply these approaches, and consider the validity of their findings in general, and in the particular context of the current UK programmes.

8.2 Posttransplant survival

The building blocks of our analysis must inevitably be the length of survival of individual patients. [1] These data are presented graphically in FIGURE 8.1. The problem in interpreting these data is that they are incomplete, in the sense that we cannot know the full survival experience of a cohort of transplant patients whilst any of them are still alive. Of the 221 patients who have received heart trans-. plants in the two programmes during the period 14th January 1979 to 30th September 1984 inclusive, 149 were still alive at 30th September 1984 and, of course, their actual future survival is unknown. In statistical terms, the data set is "censored" — that is to say at the date of data analysis there are incomplete observations of the *eventual* length of life of patients still living.

Two basically similar statistical techniques exist for estimating survival distributions with censored data; the actuarial life table method of Cutler and Ederer (1958) and the product-limit method of Kaplan and Meier (1958). Both

Figure 8.1: Posttransplant patient survival by year of transplant; Harefield and Papworth (as at 30th September 1984)

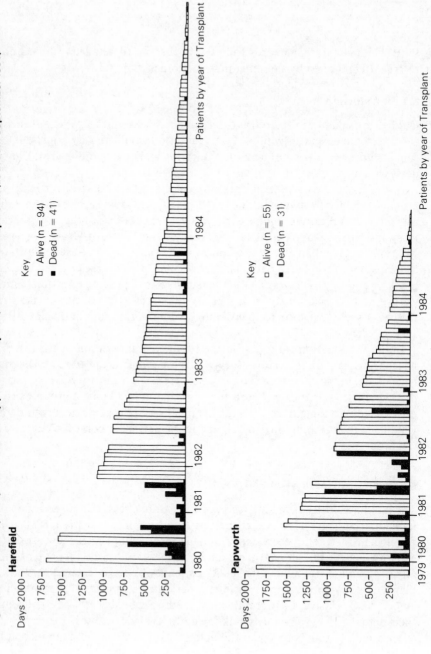

are non-parametric techniques and therefore require no assumptions about the underlying functional form of the distribution. The two methods are identical when the intervals of the life table contain, at most, one observation each. However, the discrete time product-limit estimate has the advantage of giving results that are independent of the choice of time interval.

A Kaplan-Meier product-limit survival curve is derived from survival information on all transplanted patients whether they are now dead or alive. Discrete steps down on the "curve" only occur in relation to the withdrawal of an individual from the data set by death; "losses" from the data set due to censoring are included in the calculation of probabilities in as much as the remaining population at risk is reduced. An inevitable feature of any such survival curve is that the probabilities for long-term survival (the right-hand section of the curve) are less reliable than those of short-term survival in that they are based on relatively few observations — typically those patients transplanted early in the programme. This is illustrated by the values of the standard errors which increase towards the right of the curve.

FIGURE 8.2. presents the product-limit survival curve for the two programmes combined. [2] These curves should be interpreted in conjunction with the information presented in TABLE 8.3, which summarises the cumulative survival probabilities represented by the curves for 6 months, 1 year, 2 years and 3 years after transplant with their respective standard errors. From these, confidence limits at the conventional 95% level, have been calculated for each probability estimate. It will be noted that, at each of these post-transplant intervals, the cumulative survival probabilities for the two centres are remarkably similar. The estimated survival probability for one centre is in each case well within the 95% confidence limits of the estimated survival probability of the other. The table also emphasises the small numbers of patients on which these estimates for periods in excess of one year are based.

By way of comparison, TABLE 8.4 presents survival probability for the combined UK data alongside survival probabilities from the Stanford Program. These show that taking the programmes as a whole, the UK survival experience is at least equal to that of Stanford, although it should be recognised that they cover different time periods.

Various analyses of the Stanford data have indicated significant improvements in post transplant survival probabilities since the programme started. Pennock et al (1982) report that the one year survival probability increased from 0.22 in 1968 to 0.67 in 1979. It is argued that this increase reflects a variety of changes in early post operative management. A recent important change has been the introduction of the immunosuppressive drug Cyclosporin A (CyA) used on all patients at Stanford since December 1980. Their analysis of the survival of their patients who have received CyA up to 27 September 1984 shows a one year survival probability of 0.82 (SE = 0.037). [3]

We have carried out some initial analyses to test whether or not survival rates are improving in the UK:

(A) To formally confirm that there is no significant difference between the two centres, non-parametric tests of *overall* differences in the two survival curves have been carried out. The first test (as proposed by Mantel [1966]is a generalised Savage statistic based on an exponential scores test. The second (as proposed by Breslow [1970] is analogous to the Kruskal-Wallis or generalised

71

Figure 8.2: Product-limit posttransplant survival curve for Harefield and Papworth combined (as at 30th September 1984)

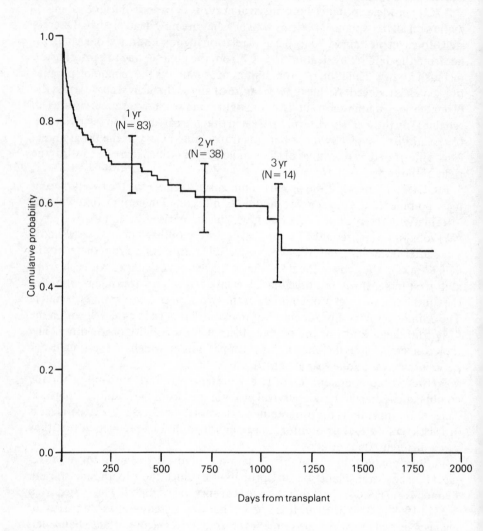

Table 8.3   Post transplant patient survival at 30th September 1984 cumulative probabilities and confidence limits

	Cumulative Probability	Standard Error	95% Confidence Limits	Number of Patients at Risk
Combined (N = 221)				
6 Months	0.7320	0.0312	(0.6708–0.7932)	115
1 Year	0.6906	0.0337	(0.6245–0.7567)	83
2 Years	0.6112	0.0416	(0.5297–0.6927)	38
3 Years	0.5218	0.0607	(0.4028–0.6408)	14
Harefield (N = 135)				
6 Months	0.7354	0.0400	(0.6570–0.8138)	65
1 Year	0.6983	0.0433	(0.6550–0.7832)	45
2 Years	0.5767	0.0626	(0.4540–0.6994)	16
3 Years	0.5767	0.0626	(0.4540–0.6994)	3
Papworth (N = 86)				
6 Months	0.7277	0.0498	(0.6301–0.8253)	50
1 Year	0.6808	0.0535	(0.5759–0.7857)	38
2 Years	0.6407	0.0574	(0.5282–0.7532)	22
3 Years	0.5082	0.0822	(0.3471–0.6693)	11

Wilcoxon test. The tests differ in the way the observations are weighted. "The Breslow test gives greater weight to early observations and is less sensitive to late events which occur when few patients on the study remain alive. Both tests are valid in large samples whether the censoring patterns are equal or unequal" (Dixon [1983]. As TABLE 8.5 (A) shows both these tests clearly suggest that we cannot reject the null hypothesis that the survival curves are sampled from the same statistical population, or in other words that the Harefield and Papworth survival probability curves are not statistically different at conventional levels of probability.

Table 8.4   Post-transplant patient survival: U.K. and Stanford experience

	Harefield and Papworth combined (1979–1984) N = 221		Stanford (1968–1984) N = 315	
	Cumulative Probability	95% Confidence Limits	Cumulative Probability	95% Confidence Limits
1 Year	0.6906	(0.6245–0.7567)	0.65	(0.595–0.705)
2 Year	0.6112	(0.5297–0.6927)	0.57	(0.513–0.627)
3 Year	0.5218	(0.4028–0.6408)	0.51	(0.449–0.571)

(B) To test for a difference in survival probabilities between the earlier and later parts of the programme we divided the combined survival data (221 transplanted patients) into two groups on the basis of the arbitrary distinction of whether the operation was performed before (N = 88) or after 1st January 1983 (N = 133). The problem of censored data for such a relatively short programme makes it very difficult to make any firm statements about changes in longer-term survival; there have been only 21 deaths in the second group of 133 patients compared with 51 deaths in the first 88 patients. The same two non-parametric statistical tests were carried out to compare the overall survival curves in the two time periods [see TABLE 8.5 (B)]. These suggest that at conventional levels of probability, there is evidence that survival has improved over time. The survival curves for the two time periods are presented in FIGURE 8.6.

(C) Cyclosporin A is now being routinely used in both UK programmes. Use of CyA began in March 1982 at Papworth and September 1982 at Harefield. Such recent introduction makes it difficult to disentangle the effect of the drug from a possible independent time trend in survival. However, as an initial analysis the posttransplant survival data were grouped in terms of pre and post introduction of CyA and tested for statistical difference between the survival curves [see TABLE 8.5 (C)]. Again using the combined data, the results suggest that we can be 99% confident in rejecting the hypothesis that pre and post CyA survival is the same, ie there is a statistical difference between the curves. The two curves are presented for comparison in FIGURE 8.7. It is interesting to note that the combined one year survival rate for the 154 patients who have received CyA is 0.8040 (SE = 0.0336); very similar to the Stanford rate reported above.

Table 8.5   Post transplant survival: Summary table of statistical differences between patient groups, as at 30th September 1984; data for Harefield and Papworth combined

	Generalised Wilcoxon		Generalised Savage	
Sub-Group	Statistic	P Value	Statistic	P Value
(A) *Hospital*: Harefield (N = 135) Papworth (N = 86)	< 0.01	0.947	< 0.01	0.953
(B) *Time*: Pre 1 Jan 1983 (N = 88) Post 1 Jan 1983 (N = 133)	13.34	< 0.001	17.36	< 0.001
(C) *Cyclosporin A*: Pre CYA (N = 67) Post CYA (N = 154)	10.65	0.001	15.34	< 0.001
(D) *Diagnosis*: IHD (N = 133) CM (N = 74)	2.06	0.152	1.15	0.283
(E) *Age*: ≤ 46 years (N = 132) > 46 years (N = 89)	0.06	0.804	0.11	0.743
(F) *Transplant sex*: Male (N = 205) Female (N = 16)	0.94	0.332	0.20	0.655
(G) *Donor sex*: Male (N = 156) Female (N = 53)	0.77	0.381	0.17	0.680
(H) *Donor age*: ≤ 30 years (N = 165) > 30 years (N = 43)	3.67	0.055	4.48	0.034
(I) *Previous Cardiac Surgery* Yes (N = 55) No (N = 157)	< 0.01	0.988	0.51	0.475

(D) Within the population of post transplant patients the survival of other distinct groups of patients can be compared. The transplanted patients were grouped by the two main diagnostic categories of Ischaemic Heart Disease

Figure 8.6: Product-limit posttransplant survival curves for combined Harefield and Papworth data by time periods (as at 30th September 1984)

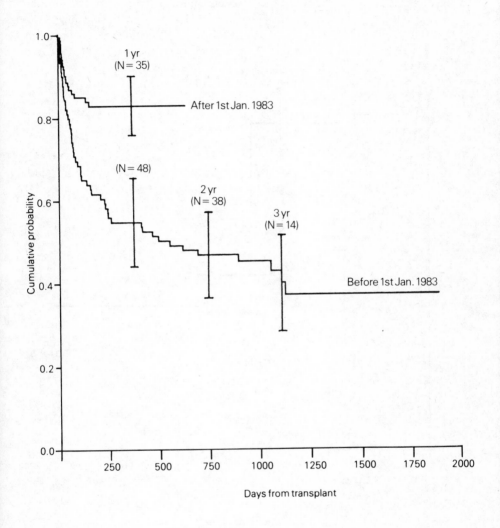

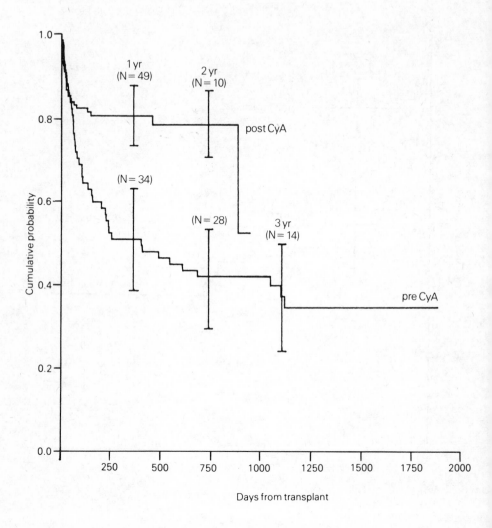

Figure 8.7: Product-limit posttransplant survival curves for combined Harefield and Papworth data; grouped by pre and post introduction of cyclosporin A (as at 30th September 19

(IHD) (N = 133) and Cardiomyopathy (CM) (N = 74) in order to compare their survival experience. (The remaining 14 "other" diagnoses were excluded in this analysis.) As TABLE 8.5 (D) indicates, no significant difference between the survival experience of the diagnostic groups could be detected.

(E) An analysis of Stanford data by Kalbfleisch and Prentice [1980[produced interesting results when examining the age of patients at time of transplant. Their study suggests that the "critical" age for transplant patients is about 46 years; "older" patients survive the operation less well. In order to examine "age at transplant" as a prognostic indicator, the combined UK transplanted patient data were split into two groups with a cut-off at 46 years; 60 per cent being "46 or less" and 40 per cent being "47 or over". No significant difference in survival between the two age groups could be detected [see TABLE 8.5 (E)].

(F) Transplants were also grouped by sex. The main problem with this comparison is that at 30th September 1984 a total of only 16 females have received heart transplants. TABLE 8.5(F) indicates that in the combined data there is not significant difference between the sexes.

(G) When transplanted patients are grouped by sex of *donor* no significant difference in transplant survival was found between male and female donors [see TABLE 8.5(G)].

(H) It seems that the age of the donor does have an effect however. The transplanted patients were divided into two groups on the basis of the arbitrary distinction of whether the donor was older than 30 years. The "older" donor group is associated with shorter survival, the difference is significant (P< 0.05). [See TABLE 8.5(H) and FIGURE 8.8.]

(I) In a number of cases, patients accepted for transplant may have undergone previous cardiac surgery. The transplanted patients were grouped, irrespective of diagnosis, by those who had and those who had not undergone previous surgery. No significant difference could be found between the two groups in terms of their posttransplant survival experience [see TABLE 8.5 (I)].

8.3 Multivariate analysis of posttransplant survival

Despite relatively well defined patient selection criteria for cardiac transplantation, it is clearly unrealistic to assume that transplanted patients form a strictly homogeneous group. A number of factors which vary between transplanted patients may significantly influence survival. In the previous section our analyses were of simple univariate "grouping" of patients.

However, this approach, despite its appealing simplicity, may hide important interactions *between* variables. The aim of the *multivariate* analysis presented in this section is to determine which of the characteristics of patient and donor vary systematically with survival. This information on relative "risk factors" may be useful in improving our understanding of the complex relationship between patient selection criteria prognostic variables and survival.

If *uncensored* survival data were available then standard regression techniques could be employed with time to death (survival) as the dependent variable and such variables as age introduced as independent or "explanatory" variables. With censored data the standard regression techniques cannot be used but a multiple regression approach for use with such data has been developed by Cox [1972]. Subsequently a number of parametric and non-parametric approaches

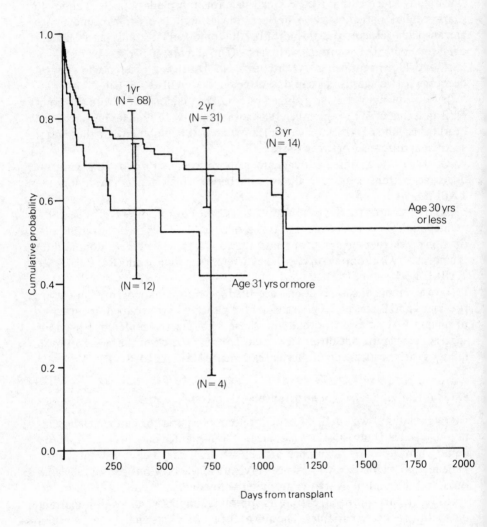

Figure 8.8: Product-limit posttransplant survival curves for combined Harefield and Papworth data; grouped by age of donor (as at 30th September 1984)

using regression techniques for analysing censored survival data have been proposed: Miller [1976]; Buckley and James [1979]; Koul, Susarla and Van Ryzin [1981]. These were recently reviewed, using Stanford Heart Transplant data, by Miller and Halpern [1982] who conclude that the "Cox partial likelihood technique" remains the most empirically reliable and theoretically valid for use with censored survival data. For a recent review of such methods see Cox and Oakes [1984].

The Cox regression technique was applied to the Stanford data by Crowley and Hu [1974], who used a variety of potential prognostic variables including: (i) age at transplant; (ii) waiting time to transplant; (iii) calendar time at transplant; (iv) previous open heart surgery; and (v) tissue mismatch. Their results and those of similar applications of covariate analysis to the Stanford data set such as that of Kalbfleisch and Prentice [1980] have been recently reviewed by Aitkin, Laird, and Francis [1983]. The general conclusions that emerge from these analyses of the Stanford data appear to be that age has relatively litle effect on survival of accepted patients before transplantation, but the posttransplant survival was significantly better amongst younger patients. Waiting time to transplant did not have a significant effect on survival. Time elapsed since the initiation of the transplantation programme had a marginally significant and positive effect on posttransplant survival (ie survival is improving over time). Previous open heart surgery seem marginally to improve pre-transplant survival. The degree of tissue mismatch, as measured by Bieber's "mismatch score", was marginally significant.

Using the same techniques as Crowley and Hu [1974], we have analysed some of the available patient variables to test whether any one or group of characteristics are useful prognostic indicators of posttransplant survival, using the Cox proportional hazards regression model — a technique which presumes that death rates may be modelled as log-linear functions of the available covariates.

Unfortunately, for some patients information on some variables is missing which slightly reduces the number of cases for analysis. We set out below (with the coding used for analysis) the discrete or continuous variables which were available for analysis and which we hypothesised might be expected to effect survival:

Covariates

WAIT	(Z0)	Waiting time from definite acceptance on programme to transplant operation (days)
AGETX	(Z1)	Age of recipient (years) at time of transplant
SEXTX	(Z2)	Sex of transplant recipient: 0 = male, 1 = female
DIAG	(Z3)	Recipient Diagnosis: 0 = Ischaemic Heart Disease, 1 = Cardiomyopathy, 2 = Other
CYA	(Z4)	Transplant immunosuppression: 0 = prior to Cyclosporin, 1 = Cyclosporin A
SURG	(Z5)	Whether recipient had undergone any previous cardiac surgery: 0 = No, 1 = Yes
TXTYPE	(Z6)	Transplant operation type; 0 = Orthotopic, 1 = Heterotopic ("piggyback")
DONAGE	(Z7)	Age of donor (years)
DONSEX	(Z8)	Sex of donor: 0 = Male, 1 = Female

79

ISCT	(Z9)	Ischaemic time of donor heart (hours)
HOSP	(Z10)	Hospital of transplant: 0 = Harefield, 1 = Papworth
CALEND	(Z11)	Calendar time in days from 1st January 1979 to time of transplant

The particular computational technique for applying the Cox regression was that of stepwise backward elimination. Originally all the variables are "forced" into the equation. At each step the variable with the poorest predictive power is eliminated. The process stops when a pre-specified significance level for coefficients is reached. The results of this technique are shown in TABLE 8.9.

When interpreting the coefficients on the independent variables, it must be remembered that the independent variable is based on death rates and is therefore *inversely* related to survival. The P values reported are "two-tailed", since we make no a *priori* assumptions about the direction of influence of any particular variable. Waiting time to transplant (WAIT) has the weakest "explanatory" power of the included variables and is the first to be eliminated from the equation. Suprisingly, the age of the recipient appears not to be significantly related to survival (P> 0.05). Nor are (at the same level of significance) the type of transplant (TXTYPE), the sex of the donor (DONSEX), the Ischaemic time (ISCT), the centre at which the transplant was performed (HOSP) or the sex of the recipient (SEXTX) or previous cardiac surgery (SURG). Recipient diagnosis (DIAG) is marginally significant (0.05 < P< 0.1) suggesting that cardiomyopathies may have poorer survival. The greatest predictive power is attributable to the CYA and DONAGE variables. There appears to be a significant (P< 0.05) inverse relationship between transplant survival and the age of the donor. Patients who have received Cyclosporin A appear to be significantly (P< 0.01) less at risk than those patients transplanted prior to the introduction of the drug. However there is a high degree of positive collinearity between the time trend variable (CALEND) and the CYA variable (r = 0.85), and the CYA variable only becomes significant when CALEND is eliminated from the equation. To test whether a time trend independent of CYA exists the data were split into the pre and post Cyclosporin periods and the same analysis run. For both groups of data TABLE 8.10 presents the stepwise procedure in summary, presenting only the initial and final equations. Prior to the introduction of CyA no independent time trend can be detected; the only significant (P< 0.05) variable influencing survival appears to be whether the patient had undergone previous cardiac surgery (SURG). After the introduction of CyA survival appears to be significantly shorter in patients who wait relatively longer for transplant (WAIT) and who receive hearts from older donors (DONAGE). However the post CyA equations must be interpreted with caution as they are based on only 24 deaths from 123 observations. Overall the evidence suggests a small but non-significant (P> 0.1) upward time trend in survival after the introduction of CyA; but the majority of the improvement in survival from the start of the programmes appears to be attributable to the introduction of CyA.

8.4 Comparative survival

The analysis of post transplant survival probabilities and risk factors does not address the issue of the extent to which cardiac transplantation affects patient

Dependent variable = log of hazards

Equation No.:	WAIT Z0	AGETX Z1	SEXTX Z2	DIAG Z3	CYA Z4	SURG Z5	TXTYPE Z6	DONAGE Z7	DONSEX Z8	ISCT Z9	HOSP Z10	CALEND Z11	
(0) beta	0.0004	0.005	-0.685	0.503	-0.664	0.455	0.500	0.043 *	-0.165	-0.235	0.265	-0.003	chi-square = 23.64 d.f. = 12
t	0.22	0.31	-1.11	1.58	-1.13	1.49	0.81	2.33	-0.55	-0.98	0.69	-0.51	p = 0.02
(1) beta	0.006		-0.694	0.488	-0.692	0.452	0.509	0.042 *	-0.171	-0.232	0.294	-0.0002	chi-square = 23.63 d.f. = 11
t	0.34		-1.12	1.57	-1.21	1.48	0.82	2.32	-0.56	-0.96	0.82	-0.47	p = 0.01
(2) beta			-0.726	0.456	-0.668	0.445	0.513	0.043 *	-0.177	-0.227	0.259	-0.0003	chi-square = 23.45 d.f. = 10
t			-1.18	1.54	-1.17	1.47	0.83	2.42	-0.58	-0.95	0.76	-0.49	p = 0.009
(3) beta			-0.741	0.461	-0.909 **	0.448	0.575	0.043 *	-0.203	-0.252	0.319		chi-square = 22.83 d.f. = 9
t			-1.21	1.55	-3.07	1.48	0.95	2.41	-0.68	-1.08	1.00		p = 0.007
(4) beta			-0.699	0.457	-0.877 **	0.436	0.511	0.041 *		-0.240	0.295		chi-square = 22.21 d.f. = 8
t			-1.14	1.55	-3.00	1.44	0.86	2.34		-1.04	0.94		p = 0.005
(5) beta			-0.694	0.448	-0.809 **	0.415		0.040 *		-0.206	0.215		chi-square = 21.56 d.f. = 7
t			-1.14	1.52	2.91	1.38		2.26		-0.91	0.72		p = 0.003
(6) beta			-0.693	0.493	-0.816 **	0.419		0.039 *		-0.142			chi-square = 21.33 d.f. = 6
t			-1.13	1.69	-2.92	1.39		2.21		-0.70			p = 0.002
(7) beta			-0.696	0.479	-0.855 **	0.398		0.041 *					chi-square = 20.57 d.f. = 5
t			-1.14	1.65	-3.12	1.33		2.35					p = 0.001
(8) beta				0.381	-0.853 **	0.392		0.039 *					chi-square = 19.41 d.f. = 4
t				1.34	-3.12	1.31		2.23					p = 0.0007
(9) beta				0.269	-0.869 **			0.039 *					chi-square = 17.70 d.f. = 3
t				1.01	-3.19			2.27					p = 0.0005
(10) beta					-0.842 **			0.039 *					chi-square = 16.62 d.f. = 2
t					-3.11			2.29					p = 0.002

** Indicates p < 0.01 (two-tailed test)
* Indicates p < 0.05 (two-tailed test)

Table 8.10 Cox regression on (1) Transplanted patients who did not receive cyclosporin A (N = 58)
(2) Transplanted patients who did receive cyclosporin A (N = 123)
Dependent variable = log of hazards

	WAIT $Z0$	AGETX $Z1$	SEXTX $Z2$	DIAG $Z3$	SURG $Z5$	TXTYPE† $Z6$	DONAGE $Z7$	DONSEX $Z8$	ISCT 9	HOSP $Z10$	CALEND $Z11$	
PRE-CYA												
Equation No.:												
(0) beta	−0.003	−0.007	−0.684	0.375	0.813*		0.031	−0.590	−0.057	0.444	0.0004	chi-square = 10.66 d.f. = 10
t	−1.08	−0.33	−0.82	0.84	2.08		1.08	−1.51	−0.14	0.76	0.47	p = 0.38
(8) beta				0.509	0.797*							chi-square = 5.56 d.f. = 2
t				1.36	2.22							p = 0.06
POST-CYA												
(0) beta	0.004	0.017	−0.492	0.330	−0.769	0.320	0.039*	0.414	−0.394	0.45	−0.0009	chi-square = 14.17 d.f. = 11
t	1.55	0.50	−1.21	1.55	1.48	0.95	2.41	−0.68	−1.08	1.00	−0.95	p = 0.22
(8) beta	0.005*				−0.916		0.056*					chi-square = 8.68 d.f. = 3
t	2.11				−1.14		2.03					p = 0.03

** Indicates $p < 0.01$ (two-tailed test)
* Indicates $p < 0.05$ (two-tailed test)
† Pre-CyA no patient, diagnosed as CM or IHD, received a heterotopic transplant.

prognosis. Clearly the fundamental question is how much longer do transplant patients live than they would have done without a transplant? It is the surgeons' judgement that each patient at the point of definite acceptance has a very poor prognosis, and is not expected to survive more than about six to twelve months without transplant. If this judgement is right with respect to the transplant group as a whole, then on average, survival in excess of that range would represent a net gain from the procedure.

The question is whether this judgement can be supported by statistical analysis of the available data. In the absence of the randomised control group, can any clinically and statistically valid inferences be drawn about the effect of transplantation on survival?

Numerous statistical analyses have been carried out on early data from the Stanford Program. It is illuminating to rehearse briefly the major comparisons that have been made, and to attempt to elucidate in an essentially non-technical way the primary problems involved and their implications for any conclusions that might be drawn from the results of the studies.

Messmer *et al* [1969], and Clark *et al* [1971], working on very early data from the heart transplant programmes at Houston and at Stanford respectively, approached the problem in similar ways. Given the stringent criteria surrounding patient acceptance onto the programmes, they considered it reasonable to assume that those patients who were accepted, but who did not receive transplants (because no suitable donor became available before they died *or* who were still waiting at the time of data collection), could be used as a comparison or approximate control group for those patients actually transplanted. It was appreciated that it was a questionable assumption that all patients accepted form an entirely homogeneous group in terms of "severity" of illness and predicted life expectancy. But making this assumption allowed the two studies to compare the survival curves of those transplanted with those for whom a donor heart was not available, in order to determine whether transplantation extended survival.

Clark *et al* compared survival from transplant operation with survival of the untransplanted from the point of *acceptance* onto the programme. Messmer *et al* included the waiting time to transplant and viewed survival for both groups of patients from their point of acceptance onto the programme. Both studies concluded that, for the particular sets of patients being analysed, transplantation appeared to increase survival in suitably selected patients.

The comparison made by Clark *et al*, continues to be presented frequently in the clinical literature, at least in the informal terms of the placing of the two curves on the same graph (for example in Jamieson *et al* [1979]; Pennock *et al* [1982]; and Reitz and Stinson [1982]. Indeed the recent Report from the Council of the British Cardiac Society (British Cardiac Society [1984]) perpetuates this spurious comparison. We stress that this comparison is *seriously misleading* as an indication of the effect of transplantation.

Gail [1972] doubted the validity of this type of comparison, and questioned whether the difference in survival between the transplanted and the non-transplanted patients is the positive result of the treatment, or simply reflects bias in the assignment of subjects to the transplanted or non-transplanted groups. His basic argument was that in both the early studies, the patient was assigned to the non-transplant group by default. The non-transplant group cannot be considered as a fair control group since the principal reason a trans-

83

plant candidate does not receive a heart is that he does before a donor can be found. Gail hypothesized that the waiting period tended to filter out the "bad risks". Gail effectively summarises his criticisms as follows:

(1) "The survival time of the non-transplanted group is shorter than would have been observed with a random assignment method, because the method used assigns an unfair proportion of the sicker patients to this group (bias)."

(2) "The survival time of the transplanted group is no longer than would have been observed with a random assignment method for two reasons. First, an unfairly large number of good-risk patients have been assigned to this group, introducing a bias. Second, the patients in this group are guaranteed (by definition) to have survived at least until a donor was available, and this grace period has been implicitly added into the survival time of the transplanted group."

Gail concluded that both Messmer and Clark in analysing data from the early programmes had over-estimated the effect of transplantation on survival. He argued that the "true increase" in survival would be that observed if the original pool of potential recipients had been *randomly* assigned to the transplantation and non-transplantation groups at the outset. He argued that the only solution to the problem of patient group assignment bias was some form of randomised controlled trail (RCT).

Suffice it to say that such an approach has not been considered acceptable here in the UK nor elsewhere. In the absence of data from an RCT, Turnbull, Brown and Hu [1974] proposed an alternative general approach to avoid the so-called "time-to-treatment" bias that Gail had identified. This was to take as the comparison group *all those patients firmly accepted onto the transplant programme*. A patient would leave this group either as a death while waiting for transplant or as a censored observation. These censored observations, or "losses" as the statistical literature also terms them, would consist of a combination of those who are: (i) still alive and awaiting transplant at the time of data analysis; (ii) any patients who were "de-selected" from the waiting list; and (iii) those who have received a transplant. With this approach, Turnbull and colleagues attempted to test the null hypothesis that heart transplantation has no effect on survival time. Their first step was to estimate what would be the distribution of survival time of *all patients accepted* if none were transplanted, using transplanted patient data as "losses" to the data-set at the time of transplant. This survivorship function can then be used to test whether the *actual* survival of *transplanted patients* is significantly different from the produced or *expected* survival, using various parametric and non-parametric tests. Their results in the context of the Stanford data were still not definitive. They concluded that, "all evaluations suggest at least a slight improvement in prognosis", but the rejection or otherwise of the null hypothesis depended crucially on the assumptions about the censored data within their survivorship function. "Without additional data on the long-term prognosis for survival for the (accepted) patient who does not receive a heart, the matter will remain in doubt."

The Actuarial Prediction Test was one simple non-parametric test used by Turnbull *et al* to compare the actual with the expected survival of transplanted patients from acceptance, so avoiding the time to treatment bias. This test was applied to the data from both UK programmes, based on *all* pre transplant survival from the point of acceptance on the programme. When (if) a patient is transplanted he becomes a loss to follow-up (censored) at that time. The hypothesis to be tested is that the *actual* number of transplanted patients who are alive now (at time of study) is no different from the number we would *expect* to be alive based on the survival experience of non (or pre) transplanted patients.

Effectively it recognises that the acceptance to transplant survival of patients who are eventually transplanted is a valid component of non-transplant survival. Every transplanted patient contributes to the non-transplanted group survival between his acceptance and transplant. It is this component that the comparisons of Messmer (1969) and Clark *et al* (1971) had ignored.

Applying the Actuarial Prediction Test to the UK data the following results are obtained:

		Harefield	Papworth
Observed number of survivals at 30th September 1984	=	94	55
Expected number of survivals	=	50.77	43.37
Variance of number of survivals	=	15.01	8.77

Thus at 30th September 1984, 94 transplanted patients from Harefield were still alive compared with the conditional expectation of 50.77 survivors without transplant, and 55 compared with 43.37 for Papworth. At each centre the differences between *observed* and *expected* survival is significant ($P < 0.01$) and the test therefore rejects the null hypothesis in favour of the alternative that survival of transplanted patients is greater than would be expected without transplant.[4]

When applied to the Stanford data it was noted that the main weakness with the Actuarial Prediction Test was that the Kaplan-Meier survivorship curve for the non (and pre) transplant experience was based on very few observations past 90 days, because few patients waited longer than that for a donor heart.

Using data from the two UK programmes combined, FIGURE 8.11 is based on 321 accepted patients: 221 become censored observations at time of transplant; 30 are lost to follow-up due either to deselection from the definite waiting list or due to being still alive and waiting at 30th September 1984; and 70 were deaths while awaiting transplant. At 90 days post acceptance FIGURE 8.11 is based on 69 patients surviving without transplant. This analysis suggests that there is a 0.5267 (SE = 0.0622) cumulative probability of surviving to one year without transplant.

In addition to the Actuarial Prediction Test, FIGURE 8.12 presents the valid comparison of all pre transplant survival from acceptance with the survival of transplanted patients from acceptance. Note that this comparison is not the same as that presented by Clarke *et al* (1971) or Messmer (1969); the important difference being that the "time to treatment" (waiting time) of eventually transplanted patients is included in the comparison. A statistical comparison of the two curves does indicate that the survival time to death from acceptance of transplanted patients is significantly ($P < 0.01$) greater than the survival time from acceptance of all pre transplant and non transplant patients, reflecting the difference in long-term survival.[5]

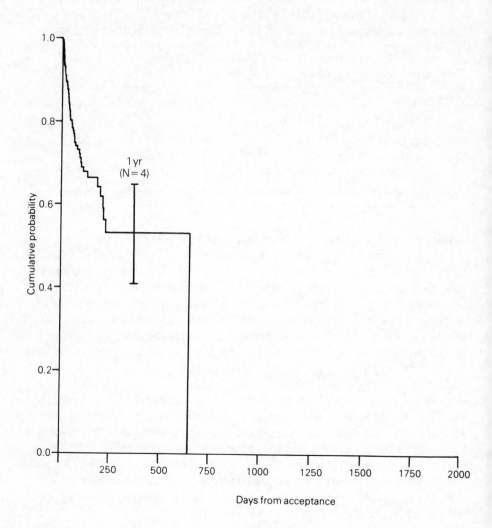

Figure 8.11 Cumulative probability of survival without transplant for accepted patients from time of acceptance, estimated from all pre-transplant experience by the product-limit method; combined Harefield and Papworth data (as at 30th September 1984)

Figure 8.12: Cumulative probability of survival without transplant from time of acceptance, estimated from all pre-transplant experience, compared with all transplanted patient survival from acceptance, combined Harefield and Papworth data (as at 30th September 1984)

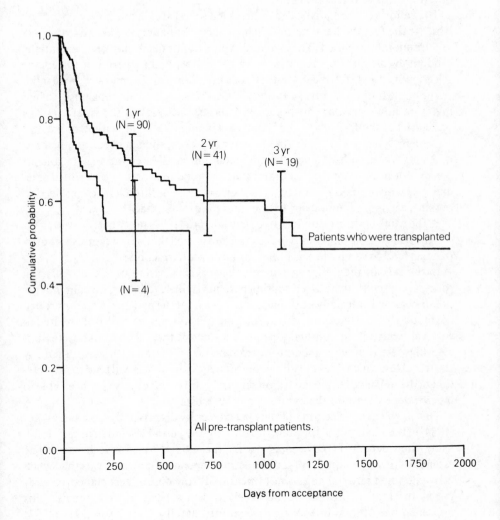

8.5 Discussion

Once the basic problem of time to treatment bias has been allowed for, a number of parametric and non parametric methods are available to test the hypothesis that transplantation increases survival time from acceptance on to the programme. But a second and more fundamental problem remains, namely the question of patient selection bias.

The validity of the statistical tests designed to test such hypotheses depends on whether the factors that determine which accepted patients receive a transplant are "random" or biased. The availability of a donor heart may be an essentially random event, but the choice of recipient is not, and if there is a systematic selection bias any statistical test that does not allow for this bias will be invalid. In the context of the Stanford Program, Gail was concerned that a positive bias might be introduced at this point by offering the heart to the fittest waiting patient. Turnbull, Brown and Hu [1974] noted that an accepted patient:

"receive a heart usually within a matter of weeks, though occasionally it has taken several months. Generally, the queue of candidates waiting for a heart consists of at most one patient, and patients receive hearts in order of queue, matched with donor on blood type, so there seems to be little chance for selection bias in assigning a donor heart to one candidate or another."

In the same Stanford context, Crowley and Hu [1977] note that:

"the belief of the physicians in the program is such that, if anything, less hardy patients tend to receive hearts preferentially over hardier ones"

In the case of the UK programmes, the surgeons assure us that any bias on their part in selection between waiting patients is likely to be negative, in that the donor heart will normally be given to the 'sickest' of the patients in any appropriate blood group. If health status at the time of transplant is positively related to survival (which is an untested assumption), and if the UK surgeons systematically bias selection of recipients towards patients of lower health status, then any statistical test which does not allow for this behavioural bias will tend to underestimate the impact of transplantation on survival. We have not so far been able to independently examine the nature of any such bias.

This problem of selection bias has been recently discussed by Cox and Oakes [1984] in their analysis of the Stanford data for the period 1967 to February 1980, using time dependent covariates within the Cox regression technique. The essence of this technique is to "define a time-dependent indicator variable which takes the value zero or one at time t (measured from date of acceptance) according as the patient has not or has received a new heart by that time". This approach was utilised previously on Stanford data by Crowley and Hu [1974] who included other fixed covariates. They conclude that, post transplant survival was significantly greater than pre transplant survival ($P = 0.01$) but this was only the case in younger patients with "good" tissue matches. The recent analysis of updated Stanford data by Cox and Oakes [1984] led them to conclude that there was "some slight evidence of a benefit from transplantation". Undoubtedly the UK heart transplant survival data is in need of further detailed analysis of this sort using combinations of fixed and time dependent covariates within the Cox proportional hazards regression technique. In particular it may be possible to further identify and quantify any potential sources of patient selection bias when allocating donor hearts and to include these as covariates in the analysis. An obvious example would be to attempt to include information from the Nottingham Health Profile at assessment as a pre transplant covariate for all accepted patients. The inclusion of such a variable might provide a way to allow for any selection bias.

8.6 Summary

All survival analyses of heart transplant patients have to cope with the fact that the data are incomplete in that the future survival of patients who are still alive is not known. Of the 221 patients who have received a transplant in the two programmes, 149 were still alive at 30th September 1984.

For the whole period of the two programmes up to 30th Setember 1984, the combined survival probabilities are 0.73 at six months, 0.69 at one year, 0.61 at two years, and 0.52 at three years. This experience is very similar to that of the programme at Stanford University Hospital and there is no significant difference between the survival probabilities from the two UK centres. It must be stressed however that the survival probabilities beyond one year are subject to broad confidence limits.

More detailed analyses of the combined Harefield and Papworth data suggest that:

—Survival has improved overtime. This is largely attributable to the introduction of Cyclosporin A.

—In terms of recipient characteristics survival does not seem to be related to age, sex their previous cardiac surgery or the type of transplant they receive. It may be infuenced by diagnosis and the length of time patients wait for transplants.

—In terms of donor characteristics, age is important: survival has been longer when hearts from younger donors were used. The donor's sex, and the length of time between donor and recipient operation do not appear to have a significant effect.

In the absence of a control group it is difficult to quantify the effect of transplantation on length of life. A number of comparisons can be made, each susceptible to possible bias. However, making the most valid comparison possible in this situation, the evidence is that transplantation significantly extends life.

Technical Notes:

[1] Throughout this chapter we refer to patient rather than graft survival. Seven patients have received a second transplant. It is their total survival from the first transplant operation that is considered. Heart-lung transplants have not been included in this survival analysis.

[2] All statistical analyses reported in this Chapter have been carried out using the BMDP Statistical Package (April 1982 Version) as installed at the University of London Computing Centre, unless otherwise stated. The computational techniques cannot accommodate a death occuring on the day of transplant. Therefore, following convention, it has been necessary to assume that in such cases the patient survived until day one.

[3] This analysis was based on 115 patients who received CyA between December 15th 1980 and September 27th 1984.

	cumulative probability	95% confidence interval
1 Year	0.82	(0.89−0.75)
2 Year	0.75	(0.84−0.66)
3 Year	0.68	(0.81−0.55)

[4] Actuarial Prediction Test.

Adopting Turnbull's notation, consider only the (M) patients who have received transplants. For patient j in this group define $Vj = 1$ if he is still alive at the time of data analysis (30th September 1984) and 0 otherwise. (ie $\sum_i^m Vj =$ actual number of survivals observed). The conditional probability that the patient j would survive to 30th September 1984 (a total of Uj days after acceptance), *given that he survived to the day of transplant* (Yj days after acceptance), is equal to the conditional expected value of Vj. Under the null hypothesis this is given by the ratio $S(Uj)/S(Yj) = Pj$, say, where the function $\hat{S}(t)$ is the Kaplan-Meier survivorship curve which gives the cumulative probability of survival without transplant. (For the combined data this is illustrated in FIGURE 8.11.)

The following results were obtained:

			Harefield	*Papworth*
Observed number of survivals $= \sum_i^m Vj$		=	94	55
Expected number of survivals $= \sum_i^m Pj$		=	50.77	43.37
Variance of survivals $= \sum_i^m Pj\,(1-Pj)$		=	15.01	8.77

The standard normal test statistic is then

$$\frac{\sum_i^m Vj - \sum_i^m Pj}{\sqrt{\sum_i^m Pj\,(1-Pj)}}$$

	=	11.15	3.93
		(P< 0.01)	(P< 0.01)

[5] Testing the hypothesis that the survival curves are from the same population the following statistics were computed:

COMBINED:

Generalised Wilcoxon	= 22.83	DF = 1	P value < 0.01
Generalised Savage	= 19.08	DF = 1	P value < 0.01

9. Quality of Life: The Nottingham Health Profile

9.1 Introduction

Alongside survival as a measure of patient benefit it is essential to consider quality of life. Improved quality has been noted in many of the accounts of the heart transplant programmes in the UK and elsewhere. These statements about changes have tended to rely on clinical judgement, unstructured patient comments, or partial measures such as return to work.

In this study we have adopted a dual approach to the identification and measurement of quality of life. To provide quantitative measures of health status and changes in them, and to permit formal comparisons, we used the Nottingham Health Profile — a fairly widely tested and utilised formal instrument for measuring patients' subjective perceptions of their health state. The statistical analysis of these results forms the basis of this Chapter. In addition however, to provide a more detailed albeit impressionistic picture of the effects of their health states on their lives before and after transplant, we carried out a series of in-depth semi-structured interviews with patients. These form the basis of Chapter 10.

9.2 The criteria for choice of the instrument to measure quality of life

Various published reports of heart transplant programmes have referred to changes in quality of life. English, Cory-Pearce and McGregor [1982] state that "the quality of life of the 14 survivors" who at the time of writing had been discharged from Papworth Hospital "has greatly improved, and most of the heart recipients are delighted with the degree of rehabilitation they have attained". Similarly Pennock et al [1982] reporting the Stanford experience stress the importance of the quality of life of surviving recipients, focussing particularly on rehabilitation "defined simply as restoration of overall functional capacity sufficient to provide the patient with an unrestricted option to return to active employment or an activity of choice."

Other studies have concentrated on the impact on the patients' family, in particular developing the work of Dr Roberta Simmons at the University of Minnesota in the context of renal transplantation. (See for example — Simmons, Klein and Simmons [1977]). The National Heart Transplantation Study in the U.S.A. (funded by the Office of Research and Demonstrations of the Health Care Financing Administration, Department of Health and Human Services) has been developing a detailed questionnaire for use with the families of transplant patients focussing particularly on the effects of the operation on family relationships (Evans, [1982b]).

Whilst recognising the importance both of return to active work and of the impact on the family as measures of particular aspects of quality of life, we were concerned to adopt an existing well validated instrument as a basic measure that would provide a more general indicator of the patients' health status.

Apart from the usual constraints of available research resources, two related factors limited our scope in deciding how to measure benefits. Firstly, there was a pressing need to ensure that the method we adopted for measuring benefits could be put into operation within a very short period after the start of the study. Secondly, the programmes were expected to involve a fairly small number of actual transplant cases. It was anticipated that there might be approximately 15 – 20 transplants per year at each centre. For both these reasons it was essential that we minimised any delay in beginning to measure the "quality of life" of patients.

But in deciding on an appropriate instrument we were once again struck by the grave imbalance between the massive volume of literature stressing the importance of using health status measures in evaluative research, and the handful of even partially acceptable instruments that had actually been developed for such measurement to the point where they could be immediately applied. Bergner et al [1976a] suggested that, "from the perspective of those assigned the task of evaluating health programmes, the greatest impediments to effective evaluation are the lack of professional consensus as to what constitutes an appropriate outcome measure and the concern that cultural differences among individuals and groups may yield problematic results when a single measure is used with a diverse population." It is still a major impediment, although some instruments do now exist.

It is not relevant to this report to attempt systematically to review the literature, particularly the vast number of conceptual and theoretical papers on principles and practices of measuring health status/quality of life. Many useful surveys already exist including: Culyer, Lavers and Williams [1971]; Sackett et al [1977]; Williams [1979]; Najman and Levine [1981]; Williams [1981]; Culyer [1983] and Teeling Smith [1983]. However we should state briefly why we chose to use the Nottingham Health Profile.

The literature identifies three broad conceptions of health on which individuals base their appraisal of their own health status: feeling-state, clinical, and performance (Baumann [1961]). In that our primary concern was to collect information on patients' perceptions of their own health, independently of clinical judgement, we obviously wished to avoid any approach that relied on clinical assessments or indeed any other external interpretation of health states. This effectively restricted us to feeling-state or performance conceptions.

The nature of the evaluative context of this study and resource and time constraints further limited our choice. Apart from the obvious questions of methodological soundness and empirical validity, we identified the following criteria for a subjective health measure appropriate to this study:

(a) any measure had to be sensitive to a wide range of health states, and appropriate to patients both before and after transplant;

(b) the process of assessment had to be acceptable to patients, and any questions easily and unambiguously understood;

(c) preferably, it would be possible to elicit the necessary information by post, rather than merely by direct interview;

(d) for purposes of comparison the measure should have been used, or should be likely to be used, in studies of other relevant groups;

(e) the choice had to ensure that a minimum of developmental work would be required so that the assessment of patients could be commenced as quickly as possible, and the system of collection and analysis of the data had to be consis-

92

tent with our available resources.

It was clear that criteria (d) and (e) required that we should, if at all possible, adopt an existing validated and widely used research instrument. We recognised that we had neither the time, nor the particular expertise, to construct a new instrument. Indeed, despite the obvious temptation to adapt or combine features of various instruments to tailor them to our particular circumstances, our concern for comparability with other studies meant that we had not only to adopt an existing instrument, but also use it in the same way as it had been used elsewhere.

9.3 The Nottingham Health Profile

After detailed consideration of the few instruments available, and following discussions with some of those who had been involved in their construction and use, we chose to use the Nottingham Health Profile (NHP), which had been devised by a team from the Department of Community Medicine at Nottingham University School of Medicine, with the then Social Science Research Council. It consists of two parts. Part I sets out to measure subjective health status by asking for responses to a carefully selected set of 38 simple statements relating to six dimensions of social functioning: pain; energy; physical mobility; sleep; social isolation, and emotional reactions.

The actual statements relating to each dimension and the weights applied to them are given in FIGURE 9.1. Patients are required simply to answer yes or no to each statement, "according to whether the statement applies to him or her in general at the time of completing the profile." All statements relate to limitations on activity or aspects of "distress". The weights enable a score from 0–100 to be calculated for each dimension of the Profile in discrete steps depending upon the particular statements that apply within that section. Scores of 100 in any dimension indicate that the respondent suffers from all the limitations included in that dimension of the NHP. Conversely a zero score in any or all dimensions represents an absence of distress. The process by which these statements were derived and chosen, and the calculation of the system of weights to be applied to them are summarised in McEwen [1983]. Fuller detail is available in Backett, McEwen and Hunt [1981]; Hunt, McKenna and McEwen [1982]; and McKenna, Hunt and McEwen [1981].

The devisers of the Profile stress that scores for the different dimensions should not be aggregated to give an overall score but that the scores should be presented as a "profile". Such a profile can show up subtler, more complex, changes in health state, but it does not provide a single summary index of quality of life.

Part II of the NHP relates to, "those areas of "task performance" most affected by health." It consists of seven statements, which refer to the effects of health problems on: occupation; ability to perform tasks around the home; personal relationships; sex life; social life; hobbies and holidays. In this section respondents are asked to answer "yes" to any of the activities if their present state of health is causing problems and affecting them. There are no weights for Part II and a simple count of the affirmative responses is used as a summary statistic.

The NHP has been applied to a fairly wide range of groups, some of which

93

Table 9.1 Nottingham Health Profile: Listing of statements and their weights

Physical mobility

I find it hard to reach for things	9.30
I find it hard to bend	10.57
I have trouble getting up and down stairs or steps	10.79
I find it hard to stand for long (eg at the kitchen sink, waiting for a bus)	11.20
I can only walk about indoors	11.54
I find it hard to dress myself	12.61
I need help to walk about outside (eg a walking aid or someone to support me)	12.69
I'm unable to walk at all	21.30
	100. 0

Pain

I'm in pain when going up and down stairs or steps	5.83
I'm in pain when I'm standing	8.96
I find it painful to change position	9.99
I'm in pain when I'm sitting	10.49
I'm in pain when I walk	11.22
I have pain at night	12.91
I have unbearable pain	19.74
I'm in constant pain	20.86
	100. 0

Sleep

I'm waking up in the early hours of the morning	12.57
It takes me a long time to get to sleep	16.10
I sleep badly at night	21.70
I take tablets to help me sleep	22.37
I lie awake for most of the night	27.26
	100. 0

Energy

I soon run out of energy	24.00
Everything is an effort	36.80
I am tired all the time	39.20
	100. 0

Social isolation

I'm finding it hard to get on with people	15.97
I'm finding it hard to make contact with people	19.36
I feel there is nobody I am close to	20.13
I feel lonely	22.01
I feel I am a burden to people	22.53
	100. 0

Emotional reactions

The days seem to drag	7.08
I'm feeling on edge	7.22
I have forgotten what it is like to enjoy myself	9.31
I lose my temper easily these days	9.76
Things are getting me down	10.47
I wake up feeling depressed	12.01
Worry is keeping me awake at night	13.95
I feel as if I'm losing control	13.99
I feel that life is not worth living	16.21
	100. 0

provide interesting comparisons and help to put the scores observed in this study into a broader context.

The NHP was devised from the outset as a questionnaire that could easily be administered by post. We therefore decided that we could aim to have it completed by patients at three-monthly intervals. It would first be administered by one of the researchers as part of a longer interview at initial assessment at Papworth or Harefield, and at any subsequent assessment or pre-operative admission irrespective of the elapsed time. For any patients "waiting" for transplants the questionnaire would be repeated on a postal basis at three-monthly intervals. Thus, whenever a transplant operation takes place, the recipient should have completed a questionnaire not more than three months earlier and, usually, more recently than that.

Similarly our aim was to have the NHP completed at three-monthly intervals after the date of transplant. Thus a basic three-monthly pattern applied to all patients from assessment for as long as we could obtain their co-operation. A copy of the Profile as used is included as Appendix A.

9.4 Statistical analysis of the NHP data

In accordance with the guidance given by the Nottingham group (Hunt, McKenna and McEwen [1981]) on the statistical analysis of Parts I and II of the health profile, the statistical tests used in our analysis are exclusively nonparametric. The more usual parametric tests are inappropriate because of the non-normal distributions of scores that result from the "arbitrary", and frequently recorded, limits to the range of values (0 and 100) for the dimensions of Part I, and the dichotomous (yes/no) responses to the areas in Part II.

To understand the various non-parametric tests that are available for such data it is important to clarify the distinction between related and independent samples. Related samples (repeated measures) refer to situations where, change can be studied from sequential observations for the *same individual;* appropriate tests include the Wilcoxon Matched Pairs Signed Rank Test used here for pre- and posttransplant comparisons and the Friedman two-way analysis of variance when more than two observations on a given individual are to be compared. For comparison between *independent samples* the Mann-Whitney U Test (two groups) and the Kruskal-Wallis one-way analysis of variance (three or more groups) can be used; an example of independent sample testing would be a comparison of *all* pre-transplant profiles with *all* posttransplant profiles: the disadvantage is that the independent samples would not be paired, nor necessarily equal in number. The advantage is that this approach utilises *all* the available pre-transplant and posttransplant profile data. On the other hand the obvious advantage of analysis based on *related* samples is that the impact of any treatment or event can be tested for without the need to standardise for other covariates such as sex and diagnosis, because these remain constant for the particular individuals.

In the analysis of Part II of the profile the chi-squared test can be used for independent samples. For related samples the McNemar test is used for paired data pre- and posttransplant. In addition the Cochran Q test is available for the analysis of more than two related samples. All the tests used are explained fully in Siegel [1956], and were conducted using the NPAR TESTS subprogram within the Statistical Package for the Social Sciences (SPSS) (Version 9.1). It should be noted that these non-parametric tests use rankings of the scores rather than their numerical values. Therefore, the "mean rank scores" quoted in the Tables reflect rankings, and their magnitudes are dependent upon the number of observations in the particular comparison.

9.5 The data

At September 30th 1984, a total of 1,036 completed profiles were available for analysis from the two programmes (Harefield 458, Papworth 578). Noting the warnings about the sensitivity of the results from such questionnaires to a fluent understanding of the intentionally idiomatic language they use (see for example the discussion in Patrick [1980] in the context of his anglicisation of an American instrument), this data set excluded a small number of profiles that had been completed by non-fluent English speaking patients.

As a summary representation of the data, FIGURE 9.2 shows in a graphical form the change over time within each dimension of the profile. Each histogram represents the mean scores obtained from all observations at each point of measurement both before and after transplant. This appears to suggest a single major shift to lower scores, representing an improvement in health, following transplantation. It hints at some deterioration in subjective perceived health between assessment and transplantation, but there is no obvious consistent trend after the three month posttransplant observation. However, the next section applies more rigorous tests of change over time in these data.

9.6 Analysis of NHP Part I.

9.6.1 Comparison of Profile Scores Before and After Transplantation

In carrying out more rigorous statistical tests, a combined total of 62 "before and after" heart transplant comparisons were available for analysis; the results of testing for significant difference using the Wilcoxon test are presented in TABLE 9.3. In all six dimensions of Section I of the profile the subjective health state of individuals from both hospitals combined showed significant improvement (P< 0.01). The greatest improvement between pre-transplant and post-transplant health appears to be in the dimension of physical mobility.

The "before and after" heart transplant Wilcoxon test was also performed when data were grouped by the two main diagnostic groups: ischaemic heart disease (34 pairs) and cardiomyopathy (20 pairs). As TABLE 9.4 indicates, all dimensions of section I show significant (P< 0.05) improvement in health irrespective of diagnosis group.

Although the before and after change, when using the three month post transplant scores, is statistically significant (P< 0.01) and represents an improvement in subjective health, how does the three month posttransplant patients' health compare with that of a "normal" population? TABLE 9.5 presents mean section scores of males at three months post transplant by age group alongside the male population "norms" produced by Hunt, McKenna and McEwen [1982]. (For this Table females were excluded because of the very small numbers transplanted in either of the two programmes.) Unfortunately, due to the high concentration of transplant patient profiles around the 40–50 year age band, little faith can be placed on comparisons of the few observations in other age

Figure 9.2: Nottingham Health Profile, Part I:
Mean scores for each section by three-month periods from assessement and from transplant. Combined hospital data, (numbers of observations above bars)

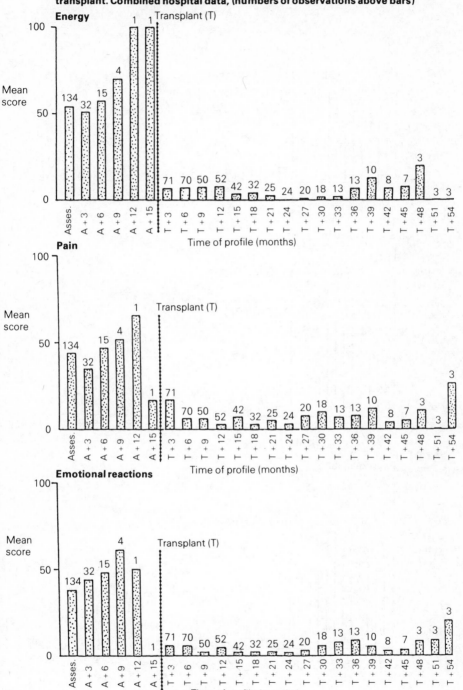

97

Figure 9.2 (continued)

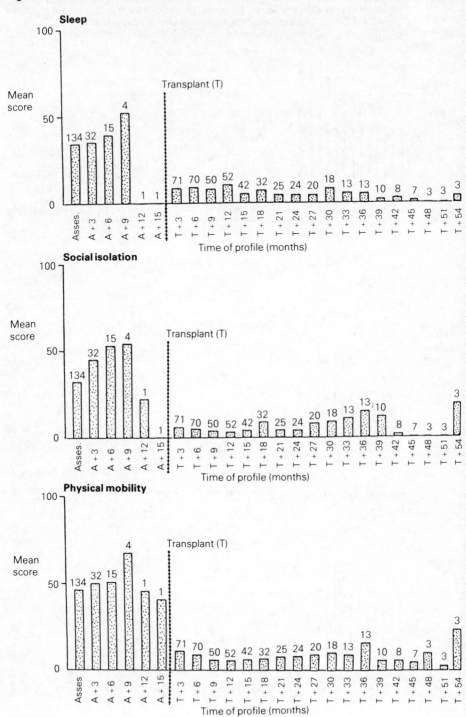

bands. Most data (n = 22) relates to the 45–49 age band; comparison with norms in this age group suggests broad similarity with normal populations except for physical mobility and social isolation where patients with transplants appear to have greater problems.

Table 9.3 **Nottingham Health Profile, Part I:**
Paired comparisons of most recent pre-transplant and three-month post-transplant patient profiles. (Wilcoxon Test)
Combined hospital data (N = 62)

	Number of ties*	Pre-transplant mean rank score	Post-transplant mean rank score	'Z' Statistic	2-Tailed P value
Energy	10	27.21	18.00	− 5.62	< 0.01
Pain	17	24.65	12.25	− 5.01	< 0.01
Emotional reactions	4	31.22	5.90	− 6.33	< 0.01
Sleep	9	30.71	11.05	− 5.36	< 0.01
Social isolation	19	23.86	3.88	− 5.52	< 0.01
Physical mobility	2	32.29	5.50	− 6.57	< 0.01

* Viz. situations in which the rank of the scores did not change.

Table 9.4 **Nottingham Health Profile, Part I:**
Paired comparisons of most recent pre-transplant and three-month post-transplant patient profiles. (Wilcoxon Test)
Combined hospital data analysed by two main diagnosis groups; Ischaemic heart disease (N = 34), Cardiomyopathy (N = 20)

	Number of ties	Pre-transplant mean rank score	Post-transplant mean rank score	'Z' Statistic	2-Tailed P value
Ischaemic heart disease:					
Energy	7	13.96	15.00	− 4.18	< 0.01
Pain	13	11.30	5.00	− 3.84	< 0.01
Emotional reactions	4	16.00	1.50	− 4.64	< 0.01
Sleep	4	17.48	5.60	− 4.21	< 0.01
Social isolation	12	12.84	3.00	− 3.82	< 0.01
Physical mobility	2	17.00	1.00	− 4.92	< 0.01
Cardiomyopathy:					
Energy	3	9.93	4.67	− 2.96	< 0.01
Pain	3	9.87	2.50	− 3.39	< 0.01
Emotional reactions	0	11.62	4.17	− 3.45	< 0.01
Sleep	4	10.17	3.50	− 2.79	< 0.01
Social isolation	6	7.88	2.50	− 3.14	< 0.01
Physical mobility	0	11.82	3.00	− 3.58	< 0.01

Table 9.5   Nottingham Health Profile, Part I:
Three months post transplant mean section scores by age group
males only combined hospital data (C), compared with normal
population males (P)

Age groups:		Energy	Pain	Emotional reaction	Sleep	Social isolation	Physical mobility
20–24	C	0	20.9	0	0	20.1	12.6
(N = 1)	P	10.1	0.7	11.6	8.4	5.5	1.5
25–29	C	0	0	5.6	0	0	0
(N = 3)	P	8.6	1.6	10.3	8.6	5.6	1.6
30–34	C	6.0	0	2.4	6.3	0	0
(N = 4)	P	4.0	2.8	6.3	6.2	2.9	1.3
35–39	C	6.0	4.3	0	3.1	0	10.7
(N = 4)	P	5.0	2.6	10.3	5.7	2.7	1.2
40–44	C	4.5	9.8	7.7	5.0	9.4	16.5
(N = 17)	P	10.1	5.8	10.4	11.9	5.0	3.2
45–49	C	8.8	6.0	6.0	8.4	6.4	13.3
(N = 22)	P	8.0	3.0	7.7	8.4	1.6	1.1
50–54	C	6.5	4.5	6.2	25.8	2.0	6.8
(N = 11)	P	11.6	7.1	10.6	13.4	5.5	4.1
55–59	C	8.0	0	0	4.2	0	3.7
(N = 3)	P	13.3	2.9	7.7	11.7	3.4	3.7

"Normal" population figures are from a total sample of 2173 randomly drawn from group general practice in the Nottingham area: Hunt, McKenna, and McEwen (1982).

9.6.2 *Change Over Time Before Transplantation*

Clearly, however, to focus attention only on a comparative static "before and after" picture of the transplant is to ignore important changes that may be occuring in subjective patient health *through time* — both before and after transplant. As noted above, the most useful test for such change is the Friedman Test for related samples. This was used to compare the pretransplant scores for individual patients definitely accepted for transplant, as recorded at assessment, three, six and nine months thereafter. No significant differences (P> 0.05) over time are indicated for any of the six dimensions. However, this test was based on only four individuals who had completed the four relevant pre-transplant profiles.

The alternative is to attempt to test the same hypothesis using independent samples and the Kruskal-Wallis one-way analysis of variance. This test (presented in TABLE 9.6) uses scores from all 187 completed pre transplant profiles (definitely accepted) at different periods following assessment. The hypothesis to be tested is that the six sets of observations relating to patients at three month periods from assessment to 15 months after assessment indicate no change over time; TABLE 9.6 indicates that this is true for all but the dimension of social isolation (P< 0.05). However, the question of *direction* of the change is difficult to answer by simple inspection of the mean rank scores. We further investigated this question using the Mann-Whitney U Test. This confirmed that the only significant (P< 0.05) changes occur in the dimension of social isolation, and indicated that there are *increases* in the mean rank score (viz deterioration in health) between assessment and three months and assessment and six months only. This is of course quite consistent with the clinical practice of trying to operate on any accepted patient who is waiting as soon as there is any further deterioration in their health.

Table 9.6   Nottingham Health Profile, Part I:
Comparison of pre-transplant mean rank scores over time;
assessment to 15 months following assessment; (Kruskal-
Wallis test) definitely accepted patients.
Combined hospital data (N = 187)

	Mean rank scores					
	Energy	Pain	Emotional reaction	Sleep	Social isolation	Physical mobility
Assessment (N = 134)	93.22	87.52	90.16	94.26	87.35	91.37
3 Months (N = 32)	87.52	107.22	99.84	95.30	108.31	98.66
6 Months (N = 15)	99.10	116.00	111.23	94.33	122.17	99.77
9 Months (N = 4)	117.38	137.75	126.00	113.38	119.13	128.00
12 Months (N = 1)	165.00	64.00	118.00	14.50	75.50	93.00
15 Months (N = 1)	165.00	64.00	10.50	14.50	22.50	75.50
Corrected Chi-Square	5.13	9.65	6.55	4.94	11.24	2.42
P Value corrected for Ties	0.4	0.9	0.26	0.4	0.04	0.78

9.6.3 *Change Over Time after Transplantation*

Applying the same framework of analysis to the posttransplant profiles, TABLE 9.7 presents results from the Freidman Test for related samples between three, six, nine and twelve months posttransplant, based on the 34 patients who had completed the NHP at all four points in time. At conventional levels of probability we cannot reject the hypothesis that, in each dimension of the profile, samples have been drawn from the same population, ie there is no evidence of change over time between the observations at three months and later observations in the first year following transplant. TABLE 9.8 applies the independent samples Kruskal-Wallis test on the same hypothesis using all 444 posttransplant profiles. It supports the view that there is no change over time. Again more detailed analysis of independent samples between three months and twelve months posttransplant using the Mann-Whitney U test has been carried out; this indicates a significant improvement in physical mobility between three months and a year, but shows no other significant change posttransplant.

Table 9.7   Nottingham Health Profile, Part I:
Comparison of mean rank scores post-transplant over time.
(Friedman Test) at 3, 6, 9, and 12 months post-transplant
combined hospital data (N = 34)

| | Mean Rank Scores | | | | | | |
	3 M	6 M	9 M	12 M	Chi-Square	D.F.	P Value
Energy	2.54	2.41	2.44	2.60	0.49	3	0.92
Pain	2.37	2.84	2.46	2.34	3.27	3	0.35
Emotional reactions	2.66	2.40	2.41	2.53	0.93	3	0.82
Sleep	2.84	2.54	2.37	2.25	4.01	3	0.26
Social isolation	2.43	2.56	2.44	2.57	0.36	3	0.95
Physical mobility	2.59	2.72	2.31	2.38	2.18	3	0.54

Table 9.8   Nottingham Health Profile, Part I:
Comparison of mean rank scores post-transplant over time.
(Kruskal–Wallis Test) at 3 to 54 months post-transplant combined
hospital data (N = 444)

| Months post transplant | | Mean rank scores | | | | | |
		Energy	Pain	Emotional reactions	Sleep	Social isolation	Physical mobility
3	(N = 71)	238.60	237.44	235.61	237.76	225.97	253.48
6	(N = 70)	227.92	231.44	235.32	226.63	225.98	230.11
9	(N = 50)	234.79	207.04	210.98	229.54	214.33	215.67
12	(N = 52)	225.28	223.44	216.81	237.13	207.13	210.53
15	(N = 42)	215.96	207.55	214.44	209.60	215.08	209.07
18	(N = 32)	205.50	195.66	202.20	217.59	235.34	214.91
21	(N = 25)	200.24	208.42	196.86	206.32	206.50	217.54
24	(N = 24)	190.50	206.17	191.19	200.42	215.19	211.35
27–30	(N = 18)	203.17	249.42	219.50	224.78	243.53	228.86
33–36	(N = 26)	217.40	247.31	248.65	221.37	258.90	240.52
39–42	(N = 18)	242.89	234.00	227.08	207.39	239.61	187.11
45–48	(N = 10)	239.20	220.30	232.35	180.85	179.00	208.20
51–54	(N = 6)	190.50	214.83	290.58	193.42	221.75	238.42
Corrected Chi-Square		16.33	11.78	13.51	8.32	12.55	11.84
P Value corrected for ties		0.18	0.46	0.33	0.76	0.40	0.46

9.6.4 *Comparison of The Assessment Populations at the Two Centres*

The preceding discussion has focussed on presenting results from the combined data from the two centres, and reflects the fact that there are very few instances in which there appear to be statistically significant differences in the existence or direction of changes in scores. However, given that two independent procedures are used to select patients for the programmes, it is interesting to compare the *levels* of scores for definitely accepted patients at assessment.

Assuming that there is no important distortion through interviewer bias or other extraneous factor, the results (presented in TABLE 9.9 using the Mann-Whitney U test) suggest that the mean scores obtained on all dimensions of Section I at assessment are significantly (P< 0.05) different between hospitals but not in a uniform direction. The scores of definitely accepted patients at Papworth indicate significantly lower subjective health in the dimensions of pain, emotional reactions, social isolation and physical mobility; patients at Harefield indicate significantly lower health in the dimensions of energy and sleep.

Another interesting point of comparison is the distinction maintained at Papworth between definite and provisional acceptance for transplant. TABLE 9.10 clearly bears out the clinical judgment on which the distinction is made: that those definitely accepted "ceteris paribus" are less healthy than those provisionally accepted. All dimensions of section I indicate significantly (P< 0.05) lower subjective health in the definitely accepted group.

Table 9.9   Nottingham Health Profile, Part I:
Comparison of mean rank scores of definitely accepted patients at assessment, by hospital. (Mann-Whitney U Test)

	Mean rank scores			
	(N = 74) Harefield	(N = 60) Papworth	Mann-Whitney 'U' statistic	2-Tailed P value corrected for ties
Energy	82.45	49.06	1113.5	< 0.01
Pain	43.59	96.98	451.0	< 0.01
Emotional reactions	60.42	76.23	1696.0	0.02
Sleep	81.77	49.90	1164.0	< 0.01
Social isolation	55.77	81.97	1352.0	< 0.01
Physical mobility	55.74	82.01	1349.5	< 0.01

9.7 Analysis of NHP Part II

The seven questions in Part II of the NHP relate to areas of life which are problematic due to health. They have no scores attached to them: the data are simply coded dichotomously as respondents answer "yes" or "no" to each question. The McNemar Test for paired comparisons was used on this dichotomous data for the latest pre transplant and three month post transplant profile, using paired samples from the same individual. TABLE 9.11 indicates that the proportion affirming that health was affecting aspects of their life fell significantly (P< 0.05) for all aspects covered. The greatest reduction would appear to be in "jobs around the home" — 82% experienced difficulty pre transplant and only 10% after it.

9.8 Discussion

The NHP has proved acceptable to patients, easy to administer by post, and fairly simple to analyse. Its questions proved understandable to (and fairly readily answerable by) patients, with perhaps the exception of Part II which some patients found very difficult to answer without qualification and explanation. Reservations can of course be raised about the validity of scores obtained. Most important perhaps is the question of whether post-transplant "euphoria" or simple gratitude for having received a transplant, lead patients to misrepresent their health state (consciously or subconsciously).

Table 9.10   Nottingham Health Profile, Part I:
Comparison of all pre-transplant mean rank scores for definitely and provisionally accepted patients at Papworth.
(Mann-Whitney U Test)

	Mean rank scores			
	(N = 90) Definite	(N = 55) Provisional	Mann-Whitney 'U' statistic	2-Tailed P value corrected for ties
Energy	85.59	52.39	1341.5	< 0.01
Pain	85.22	53.00	1375.0	< 0.01
Emotional reactions	83.45	55.90	1534.5	< 0.01
Sleep	83.12	56.45	1564.5	< 0.01
Social isolation	86.21	51.38	1286.0	< 0.01
Physical mobility	82.94	56.73	1580.0	< 0.01

Table 9.11   Nottingham Health Profile, Part II:
Paired comparisons of affirmative responses to questions pre-transplant and three months post-transplant, (McNemar Test). Combined hospital data (N = 62)

	Affirmative responses					
	Pre-transplant No.	%	3 month post transplant No.	%	Chi-Square	2 Tailed P value
Area of life:						
Occupation	33	(53)	11	(18)	20.05	< 0.01
Jobs around the home	51	(82)	6	(10)	43.02	< 0.01
Social life	54	(87)	8	(13)	42.19	< 0.01
Home life	37	(60)	1	(2)	34.03	< 0.01
Sex life	44	(71)	15	(24)	25.29	< 0.01
Hobbies	50	(81)	12	(19)	32.59	< 0.01
Holidays	53	(85)	14	(23)	35.22	< 0.01

In practice the patients' subjective judgments which underly their NHP scores, seem to correspond well with the informal expectations and views of both the researchers involved and the clinicians concerned. They are certainly supported by the results of the in-depth interivews reported in the following Chapter. Similarly the changes at an individual level seemed to be validated by the clinical judgments of their changing health states. As we have already noted, the Profile scores mirror well the independent pre-operative clinical judgments at Papworth that allocated the patients to the definite and provisional categories.

A recent study has shown how crucially the values of the weights depend upon the scaling model used and suggests that for at least one category (sleep) alternative weights are equally compatible with the original data. (Kind, 1982.) Kind's paper, using the Bradley-Terry rather than the Thurstone model to scale the weights, calculates alternative weights for just one dimension — sleep. Applying Kind's recalculated weights to the main comparisons made in this chapter leads to no substantive change in our conclusions. For example the improvement between the most recent pre transplant and the three months post transplant mean rank scores for the sleep category (shown in TABLE 9.3) is highly significant whichever of the two sets of weights are used. We further tested the sensitivity of the results in TABLE 9.3 by applying unitary weights to all the questins in each dimension. The results presented in TABLE 9.12, similarly show that thepost transplant improvement is highly significant with these alternative (arbitrary) weights.

There were however undoubtedly problems over the responses to Section II, particularly with the question relating to occupation. For example some patients unable to work because of their health recorded no problem in this respect, whilst other patients did identify a problem. More generally, it seems that other users of the Profile, and indeed those who developed it, have reservations about this section. However, most of the aspects of life covered in NHP Part II were considered in much more detail in the interviews we carried out. These are reported in the next Chapter.

Table 9.12 Nottingham Health Profile, Part I:
Sensitivity analysis using unitary weights. Paired comparisons of most recent pre-transplant and three-month post-transplant patient profiles. (Wilcoxon Test) Combined hospital data (N = 62)

	Number of ties	Pre-transplant mean rank score	Post-transplant mean rank score	'Z' statistic	2-Tailed P value
Energy	5	29.35	9.50	− 6.49	< 0.01
Pain	25	21.71	12.59	− 3.21	< 0.01
Emotional reactions	8	28.23	6.50	− 6.16	< 0.01
Sleep	11	27.36	10.00	− 5.84	< 0.01
Social isolation	22	21.91	12.50	− 4.50	< 0.01
Physical mobility	4	31.17	7.00	− 6.40	< 0.01

9.9 Summary

As a method of measuring patient benefit in terms of quality of life, we used an existing validated instrument — the Nottingham Health Profile. This measures a respondent's perception of his own health through his answers to a series of questions relating to "distress" in terms of six dimensions; — physical mobility, pain, sleep, energy, social isolation and emotional reactions. The NHP was administered to patients at assessment and then every three months prior to transplant; it was then completed every three months posttransplant. It proved easy to use and an effective instrument, and the scores based on patients' subjective perceptions in practice tallied well with independent clinical and social judgements.

The Profile scores were analysed using non-parametric statistical tests both in terms of comparisons for the same individual over time and for discrete groups of patients at different points of time.

Both forms of analysis showed significant improvement in health (or reduction of distress) when pre and posttransplant scores were compared. The posttransplant scores compared closely with those for males of the same age group from a general population.

Looking at pretransplant data there was no evidence of change over time (between assessment and transplantation). However, the expected difference between patients in the definite and provisional groups was confirmed in their NHP scores — the provisional patients being less "ill".

There was also no evidence of either systematic improvement or deterioration in health after the three month posttransplant period, by which point the patients had attained an essentially normal state of health.

10. Quality of Life: Patient Interviews

10.1 Introduction

In adopting the Nottingham Health Profile as our main instrument for "measuring" the subjective health status of patients in the transplant programme, we well recognised that this alone would be insufficient to provide a vivid and detailed picture of the implications of the patients' health for their quality of life both before and after transplantation.

The information from Part II of the NHP on the effect of their state of health (presented in chapter 9) on seven important dimensions of life provides a first indication of some of the broader aspects of "quality" but it is necessarily fairly superficial. We therefore also undertook a series of detailed interviews with patients. One member of the Research Team at each Centre carried out the interviews. A common semi-structured format and an agreed checklist of open-ended questions were used, to focus the interviews on certain topics, but the patients were encouraged to discuss the topics freely. The interviews covered the following areas:

> Work Situation
> Everyday Activities
> Hobbies and Interests
> Social Life
> Family Relationships
> Attitudes To:
> > - Illness
> > - Transplantation
> > - Hospital Check-Ups
> Quality of Life
> Disadvantages of Transplantation.

The patients were interviewed pre-operatively during their assessment period in the transplant centres, and then post-operatively at six months, one year and annual anniversaries thereafter. Normally these again took place at the transplant centres although some were conducted in the patients' homes. Typically the length of the interviews was about one hour. They were conducted during the period April 1982 until April 1984.

The evidence produced by such interviews is of a "softer" nature than the relatively "hard" data produced elsewhere in this Report. Such material is potentially subject to the well known sources of interviewer bias (Moser and Kalton [1971]). Inevitably, it is subject to a possible effect of the patient/interviewer interaction, and of errors in the responses given. Our interviewers took great care to ensure that patients understood that these interviews were not part of their assessment or review by the clinicians, and would in no way affect their assessment or continuing treatment. Their individual replies would be held in strict confidence, and would not be revealed to the clinicians.

Equally there was potential for interviewer bias, both in recording the information from the interviews, and in selecting verbatim comments from the wealth of interview material for this report. Every effort was made to ensure similar format during interviews and the choice of reported comments has been made to give as fair and accurate a picture as possible, albeit an "impressionistic painting", of the quality of life of the patients concerned. Given the small numbers of observations, we believed that the theoretical gains in accuracy from using a formalised and hence constraining questionnaire, would not justify the loss of the wealth of vivid detail that our approach in practice provided.

Nevertheless we have chosen to present the results of the interviews from the centres quite separately — not in the expectation that this would indicate any substantive differences between the two centres in the quality of life of patients before or after transplant — but rather to allow for two independent sets of impressions to be quite independently recorded. In the final event the similarity of those two sets of impressions is quite striking.

10.2 Harefield

10.2.1 Numbers of patients interviewed and their main characteristics

A total of 90 patients were interviewed at the time of their assessment for transplant. This group excludes a small number of patients too ill to be interviewed; these were usually emergency admissions from other hospitals. The outcomes of the 90 patients following interview are shown in TABLE 10.1H; as can be seen, 27 patients were given a follow-up interview post-operatively. (It was not possible to carry out a follow-up interview on one patient). Eighteen patients had been transplanted less than six months before the end of April 1984 [our cut off point for the interviews] ; five were still waiting. Twenty-nine died. Ten were, following assessment, considered unsuitable for a transplant. Of the 27 followed-up post-operatively, it was possible to interview 26 at 6 months, 16 at one year, and 4 at 2 years. In addition, 10 patients who had been transplanted prior to the research commencing, were interviewed post-operatively.

Table 10.1H   Post transplant follow up of 90 patients interviewed at assessment (Harefield)

	Number	Percent
Interviewed Posttransplant:	27	30.0%
— at six months	26	
— at one year	16	
— at two years	4	
Not Subsequently Interviewed:	63	70.0%
— transplanted in the last six months	18	
— patients still waiting for transplant	5	
— died pre-operatively	14	
— died post-operatively	15	
— rejected for transplant	6	
— received other cardiac surgery	4	
Total	90	100.0%

TABLE 10.2H shows the breakdown by the Registrar General's social classification of all the patients interviewed at assessment: 59 per cent of the patients were from non-manual classess (I,II, and IIIN) and 41 per cent were from manual classes (IIIM,IV and V). Reflecting the situation for the programme as a whole, the two main presenting diagnoses were IHD and CM. Of the patients interviewed approximately 56 per cent were suffering from ischaemic heart disease, almost all of them males, and 29 per cent were cardiomyopathies with a male to female ratio of 4:1 (TABLE 10.3H).

10.2.2 Patients at time of assessment

Work Situation

The effects of "end-stage" cardiac disease on people's ability to work and perform other everyday functions can be quite devastating, with many activities coming to an abrupt halt. Possibly the most important of these is a person's capability to work, which is usually important not only from a financial point of view but also provides a sense of independence and plays a part in family stability. Inability to work, particularly over a long period, can adversely affect these.

Table 10.2H Social class of patients interviewed at assessment (Harefield)

	Numbers by Social Class:					
	I	II	III	IV	V	Total
Manual	0	0	24	9	3	36
Non-Manual	5	36	11	0	0	52
*Total	5	36	35	9	3	88*

* Social class of two patients not known

Table 10.3H Age/sex by diagnosis for patients interviewed at assessment (Harefield)

Diagnosis	% of sample	Male: Female ratio	Average age	Age range
IHD	55.5	24:1	48	33−59
CM	28.9	4.25:1	43	26−57
Other	8.9	—	—	—
Total	93.3	9:1	45	13−59

Of the 90 patients interviewed, this section was not strictly applicable to six — (5) housewives and (1) school-child. The number of subjects working at the time of interview was only 3, with the remaining 96.4 per cent not working (see TABLE 10.4H). Of those not working, 63 per cent still had jobs kept open for them whereas 27 per cent were unemployed and nearly 10 per cent were medically retired. The high proportion of patients who were unemployed can be accounted for by the fact that many of them had lost their jobs through ill-health.

The comments made and feelings expressed by the patients about not being able to work can be grouped under various headings. Sixty-four per cent expressed adverse views about not working, 16 per cent said they missed work, and 11 per cent expressed no comment. Interestingly, about 9 per cent said they were not unhappy about not working because it was, "a rest from a previously hectic working life".

However, two-thirds expressed anger, bitterness, unhappiness, frustration and depression. Those who had adverse feelings often expressed strong emotions:

"I feel in a rage sometimes";

"I feel useless, my life is dwindling to an existence";

"horrible that I can't work, its the pressure it puts on my wife, having no money in her purse";

"now I feel like an old man";

"if I can't work, what the hell can I do?";

"after 27 years, I feel I've let myself down and the firm".

Table 10.4H: Employment position of patients interviewed at assessment (Harefield)

	Number	Percentage
Working	3	3.6
Not Working	81	96.4
— Job kept open	53	63.1
— Unemployed	23	27.4
— Medically Retired	8	9.5
Total:	84	100.0

Frustration was also expressed:

"its all this hanging about doing nothing";

"work was my life"; "since not working, I've had to learn a different way of life";

"I'm frustrated because I've still got 15 years of good work in me".

Patients also said they became depressed at their inability to work and this was linked in almost all cases with the role-reversal whereby the wife became the bread-winner:

"I feel downgraded at having to rely on my wife's pay-packet";

"because my wife works and I can't, I like to be the man of the house";

"depressed, half a man";

Less strong feelings were expressed by others:

"I miss work, I'm keen to get back, I don't like being inactive";

"I don't like lying around doing nothing";

"I'm someone who loves work".

In all, some 80 per cent of the total patients perceived the inability to work as a loss to their lives.

Everyday Activities

This section includes information on some of the common everyday things that most of us take for granted, eg walking, shopping, gardening. Walking or physical mobility is one of the most important. All manner of activities either stop, or are affected by, an inability to walk, or being able to walk for short distances only. TABLE 10.5H shows the distances that the patients estimated that they were capable of walking; as can be seen, 10 per cent could not walk at all as they were bed-ridden, over 50 per cent said they could not walk for more than 50 yards, and nearly 75 per cent could not walk for more than 100 yards. Only 11 per cent could walk for more than 400 yards. Many of the latter group were in fact deemed unsuitable for a transplant in that they were not considered to be ill enough.

Table 10.5H: Walking capability of patients interviewed at assessment (Harefield)

Distance:	Number	Percentage
Nil (Bed-ridden)	9	10.0
House-bound	13	14.4
< 50 yards	26	28.9
51–100 yards	19	21.1
101–200 yards	5	5.6
201–300 yards	1	1.1
301–400 yards	7	7.8
> 400 yards	10	11.1
Total	90	100.0

NB. All these distances are approximate judgements of the patients.

Many other everyday activities are adversely affected and these are shown in TABLE 10.6H. The heavier activities were badly affected, with 90 per cent or more in each case reporting a complete stop: shopping, gardening, painting and decorating, housework, home repairs, cleaning and maintaining a car. Those who could still manage to do some of these activities, nevertheless reported that they did them more slowly, or became tired easily.

Hobbies and Interests

Some hobbies and interests overlap with other sections, eg gardening (described within the umbrella of "everyday activities"), and some sports may overlap with social lfie. However, some arbitrary distinctions were made, mainly that a hobby or interest was seen as something chosen as an activity rather than a necessary chore such as gardening, which nevertheless may be enjoyed. Where sports participation overlapped with attending sports social clubs, the sport itself is regarded as a hobby and the socialising that goes with the sport is regarded as social life.

The range of different hobbies and interests named by the subjects was quite staggering. It was therefore decided to classify them into three groups according to their required physical activity: active, semi-active and sedentary. Using this classification 98 per cent of patients at assessment said that active interests had stopped, 86 per cent said that semi-active interests had been affected, and even 30 per cent said that sedentary interests were affected due to poor concentration or tiredness.

Social Life

Social activities had completely ceased for 81 per cent of the patients, with a further 8 per cent saying that social life was restricted, and 11 per cent who said it was not affected. Of this last group, more than half said that they had always led

111

Table 10.6H **Extent to which particular activities were reported as being limited by health amongst patients interviewed at assessment (Harefield)**

Activity:	Yes		No	
Shopping	5	(12%)	37	(88%)
Gardening	2	(3%)	70	(97%)
Painting/Decorating	6	(9%)	63	(91%)
Housework	3	(11%)	23	(89%)
Cooking	15	(54%)	13	(46%)
Home Repairs	7	(13%)	48	(87%)
Driving Car	29	(38%)	42	(62%)
Car Cleaning	3	(5%)	55	(95%)
Car Maintenance	2	(9%)	20	(91%)

a quiet social life, and spent their time with their family. Typical comments from patients were as follows:

"it's come to a full-stop";

"I can't go anywhere";

"the children don't go anywhere now. I'm stuck, so they're stuck";

"non-existent";

"I spend most of the day in bed".

Several activities, such as dances, parties, eating in restaurants, family outings and attending sports meetings, had completely stopped in approximately 95 per cent of cases. Other activities, such as visiting friends, going to the cinema or pub, had completely stopped in more than three quarters of cases. Receiving visits from family or friends was, not surprisingly, the least affected — only 30 per cent said it was affected. However, of those who said it was not affected, half had stopped giving parties or dinner-parties.

Family relationships

Family relationships may, or may not be adversely affected when one member of the family has a serious illness. In our sample, 53 per cent of patients said that relationships were not affected, with a quarter of them saying that they were even more close to their spouse because of the illness. However, 47 per cent said that the illness had affected family relations. Of these, 36 per cent said they were more short-tempered or irritable with their spouse and their children, 29 per cent with their spouse only, and 21 per cent with their children only. There were only two reported cases of the illness seriously affecting their marriages.

Attitudes

Attitudes towards the illness, the necessity for a transplant and towards donors, varied considerably. Some were in a highly emotive state or a state of shock, whereas others had already passed through these phases and had developed methods of coping with the psychological trauma of their situation. (The "coping model" described in Ray, Lindop and Gibson [1982] has been used to structure this section.)

112

(i) Attitudes to Illness

Anger as an emotion, or as a means of assertive coping, is difficult to distinguish, but for our purposes this is of little importance. Patients who felt angry or bitter about the illness made up 42 per cent of the sample, with the most common statement being: "why me?". Several patients felt angry at becoming ill because they had been very active or fit before:

"Why me? I've been fit all my life and now I feel useless".

Others wondered what they had done to deserve it:

"I consider myself a kind-hearted person and I don't deserve it. It makes me angry that my life has come to a full-stop".

Others felt unhappy and bitter:

"I've been picked out too early, I don't think I deserved it yet. I was a fit man and now, suddenly, I'm not. If it had been gradual, it would't be so bad";

"angry at being thrown on the scrap-heap and being no good to anyone".

Half of them remained angry about the illness, whereas a third coped by accepting the reality of it (resignation).

About 13 per cent of the patients recognised they were depressed:

"it's brought me down and, if there's no help, I'll give up and hope to die";

"life should be something more than just existing. I would rather die than be in this condition indefinitely";

"because I don't think I have long to live without the transplant";

I get fed-up with myself. It gets me down because I can't do what I want to do. I see others enjoying themselves, and I can't do it";

and from a 22 year old:

"people laugh at me because I'm so skinny because of the illness. I can't get clothes to fit me, and I haven't got a girlfriend".

Some 27 per cent coped with the illness by resigning themselves to it:

"it could have happened to anybody, it just happened to be me";

"I just feel it has happened and I have accepted that these things happen";

"I know that one day we all have to die";

"that's the way it is, that's life".

Small numbers coped by using avoidance:

"sometimes I feel its all a lie and I don't believe its happening";

or control:

"something has got to be done about it, knowing is the answer";

or minimisation:

"at first I didn't realise how serious it was. I wondered what was all the fuss about heart attacks".

(ii) Attitudes to Transplantation

The majority of patients (79%) had a positive attitude towards receiving a transplant:

"I want it 100 per cent";

113

"if I could have it tonight, I'd have it done";
"I feel great about it because I know that's my chance";
"hope, another chance. I see it as part of a miracle";
"I want the chance of life";
"I'm not afraid of having it, but I am afraid of not gettng it";
"I wait for it every moment";
"I accept it fully";

A few patients (17%) expressed fear about having a transplant:
"it frightened me, took my breath away";
"it worries the pants off me";
"that I may not wake up again";
"scared about it";
"its the unknown".

Even fewer patients (4%) were doubtful or worried about it:
"will it make me a useful member of society again?";
"very mixed feelings, its like sitting in a vacuum".

(iii) Attitudes to Donors

The vast majority (97%) said that they were not concerned about receiving a donor heart, although a fifth of them said they were sorry that someone had to die that they might benefit. Typical comments were:
"I carry a donor card myself, I'm prepared to give all my bits, and happy to accept other people's bits";
"its a gift";
"its sad that someone has got to die to give me a new lease of life, but why bury it, or burn it, when it can be used".

A small number (3%) did not have such a positive attitude:
"I am worried about the ethics, the right to use someone else's life to continue my own";
"I'm scared that someone has to die to help me, and scared of having someone else's heart inside me".

Quality of life

We were able to classify the patients' descriptions of their quality of life before transplant: 87 per cent said it was very bad; 13 per cent said it was neither good nor bad, but nobody said it was good. Of the majority who said their quality of life was very bad, a third of them described it as non-existent or nil:
"virtually non-existent, very, very poor";
"it's simply existing. You're alive but not living, you just exist";
"this is no life at all";
"as bad as I could imagine it, sitting in a chair in front of the window all day. Even doing that makes me breathless".

Others described it as:

"third class";
"boring";
"I feel the odd one out";
"extremely limited".

However, the small number who said it was neither good nor bad, said:
"life is precious, whatever condition you're in";
"I still enjoy life, despite the reduction";
"compared with some I could be a lot worse";
"life is sweet, even if its come to a full stop".

10.2.3   Patients posttransplant

Work Situation

Eleven of the patients (44%) had returned to work six months following the transplant. A further six (24%) still had jobs to return to when they were fit enough, and eight (32%) patients who were unemployed or medically retired before the operation remained so afterwards (see TABLE 10.7H). One year posttransplant, 12 of the patients (71%) had returned to work. A further two (12%) still had jobs kept open for them, and three (17%) had been unemployed or had retired before the illness. Two years posttransplant, three out of four patients were working: these figures contrast with the pre operative figure of 96% not working.

All of the patients who had returned to work expressed great pleasure that they were able to do so:
"tremendous, that I can now work again";
"fantastic, I missed it so much, work is really important to me";
"tremendous, to my mind this is the culmination of the operation";
"its magic".

Almost three quarters of those who remained unemployed were actively trying to find work. Several of them felt frustrated at not being able to get a job, when they felt fit enough to work.

Table 10.7H   Employment position of posttransplant patients interviewed (Harefield)

	At 6 Months		At 1 Year		At 2 Years	
	No.	%	No.	%	No.	%
Working	11	44	12	71	3	75
Not Working	14	56	5	29	1	25
Of Which:						
— Job Kept Open	6	24	2	12	—	—
— Medically Retired *	1		1		—	
		32		17		25
— Unemployed*	7		2		1	

* Unemployed or retired before
the operation

115

Everyday activities

The distances that the patients could walk, following transplantation, were vastly increased. Pre-operatively 75 per cent could not walk further than 100 yards, some were bedridden or housebound. By 6 months post-operatively, 96 per cent could walk for 1 mile or more, and nearly 40 per cent were able to walk for 5 miles or more (TABLE 10.8H). Of those interviewed at 1 year post transplant, all could walk a mile or more with half managing 5 miles or more. The trend continued and at 2 years 75 per cent were able to walk for 5 miles or more.

Everyday activities also showed considerable improvement compared with the pre-operative figures, (see TABLE 10.9H). At 6 months, the proportion of patients able to do things compared with the number (in brackets) pre operatively is as follows: shopping, 100 per cent (12%); gardening, 85 per cent (3%); painting/decorating, 77 per cent (9%); housework, 100 per cent (11%); cooking, 100 per cent (54%); home repairs, 88 per cent (13%); driving a car, 95 per cent (38%); cleaning a car, 82 per cent (5%); car maintenance, 83 per cent (9%).

This improvement continued at 1 year and at 2 years, with all of the patients (100%) who had mentioned these tasks pre-operatively, able to perform them after the transplant.

Hobbies and interests

The majority of patients were eventually able to participate in their former hobbies and interests. Not surprisingly they were slower to resume the most active interests: 68 per cent at 6 months; 95 per cent at 1 year and 100 per cent at 2 years (compared with 2 per cent pre operatively). Semi-active and sedentary interests had been resumed by all but one patient interviewed by six months.

Table 10.8H Walking distance of post operative patients at 6 months (Harefield)

	Six Months		One Year		Two Years	
Walking distance	No.	%	No.	%	No.	%
200 Yards	1	3.9	—		—	
1 Mile	1	3.9	—		—	
2 Miles	3	11.5	1	5.5	—	
3 Miles	8	30.8	5	27.8	—	
4 Miles	3	11.5	3	16.7	1	25.0
5 Miles	4	15.4	3	16.7	3	75.0
> 5 Miles	6	23.1	6	33.3	—	
Total:	26	100.0	18	100.0	4	100.0

Social life

The majority of patients were able to resume normal social lives: 95 per cent said they were back to normal, whereas 1 (5%), a young housewife, said her social life was less than before but she was quite happy, "staying at home and devoting time to my children". The vast majority of activities previously enjoyed had been resumed by the patients at six months.

116

Table 10.9H Extent to which activities that had been reported as limited by health at assessment (Table 10.6H) were unrestricted posttransplant (Harefield)

Activity	At 6 Months		At 1 Year		At 2 Years	
	Yes	No	Yes	No	Yes	No
Shopping	17 (100%)	0	11 (100%)	0	2 (100%)	0
Gardening	17 (85%)	3 (15%)	16 (100%)	0	4 (100%)	0
Painting/Decorating	13 (77%)	4 (23%)	14 (100%)	0	4 (100%)	0
Housework	6 (100%)	0	6 (100%)	0	1 (100%)	0
Cooking	9 (100%)	0	9 (100%)	0	1 (100%)	0
Home Repairs	15 (88%)	2 (12%)	13 (100%)	0	3 (100%)	0
Drive Car	19 (95%)	1 (5%)	14 (100%)	0	2 (100%)	0
Clean Car	14 (82%)	3 (18%)	13 (100%)	0	2 (100%)	0
Car Maintenance	5 (83%)	1 (17%)	4 (100%)	0	1 (100%)	0

Typical comments regarding resumption of social acitivities were:
"I can't get over the novelty of doing everything again without worrying about it";
"back to normal, no restrictions at all";
"I can take the children out at weekends again";
"very busy";
"it's increased, better than it used to be".

Family relationships

Family relationships also improved. Whereas at assessment 59 per cent had said that their family relationships were affected by their health, at one year and two years all said that their family life was now unaffected.
"there are no strains now because we don't have the fear of the illness";
"everything is normal now";
"I'm a more active member of the family now";
"it's better than it's ever been, my temper isn't as bad".

However, this improvement seems to take time as 35 per cent of patients said relationships were affected at six months post operatively. Most of them confessed to being still short-tempered or irritable with their spouses or children. Interestingly, about half attributed their short-temper to their wives trying to treat them as if they were still ill: a habit that, perhaps not too surprisingly, needed time to break.

Attitudes

(i) *Attitudes to Transplantation*

All of the patients had a positive attitude towards transplantation at all post-operative intervals. Typical comments were:
"fantastic, no regrets";
"the best thing that's happened to me in my adult life";
"it's a different way of life altogther, not living in fear of pain, fantastic";
"I'd recommend it to anyone who needed it";
"it's a bonus to open my eyes in the morning";

and in the case of one patient who received the transplant on his birthday: "the best birthday present I've ever had!".

(ii) *Attitudes to Donors*

None of the patients said that they had any problems regarding the donor. The majority expressing gratitude to the donor families for allowing the organs to be used. A few patients said they sometimes thought about the donors:
"I think about the donor at times";
"I normally don't thing about it but, as it's the anniversary, I wonder who he was and how his family are";
Some patients said they would like to meet the donor's family:
"I sometimes wonder who the donor was and would like to contact the family to thank them. Without it, I wouldn't be here".

(iii) *Attitudes to Hospital check-ups*

Regular hospital check-ups are essential for transplant patients, in order to detect possible rejection. The patients were asked about their attitude to these check-ups. At 6 months, some 88 per cent saw them as not a problem:
"they've got to be done";
"it's a routine to me";
"very grateful, I'd go every day if I had to".
A small number thought them a nuisance:
"a bit cumbersome, but necessary";
"I get a bit fed-up with it".
Over time the feelings of nuisance disappeared.

Quality of life

A complete contrast occurred between the pre-operative and post-operative groups, for whereas none of the pre-operative group said that their quality of life was good, non of the post-operative group said that it was bad. In fact, 88 per cent said that their quality of life was good, with the remainder saying that it was better than before the operation. At 1 year and at 2 years, all of the patients reported that their quality of life was good. Typical comments were:
"excellent";
"as normal";
"very good, every day is a bonus";
"I can now lead a normal life of high quality, which is just the same as before the illness. I can now do all of the things I ever could";
"marvellous, absolutely superb";
"better than it's ever been";
"it's 100 per cent again, before it was like a living death, this was my last hope";
"life is fuller and richer than before the transplant".

Disadvantages of transplantation

The patients were asked if they thought there were any disadvantages of having had the transplant. At 6 months, 88 per cent said that there were no disadvantages and 12 per cent said that there were:

"having to take drugs regularly";

"the frequent hospital check-ups";

"the extra financial hardship of returning for hospital check-ups".

However, at 1 year and at 2 years, none of the patients said that there were any disadvantages.

Typical comments were:

"I can't think of any. I lead a completely normal life, rather better than before I was ill";

"I'd be dead now, there can't be any disadvantages";

"none, I'm happy to be back to a normal life";

"I only had 4 to 6 weeks to live before the operation, so how can there be any disadvantages?"

10.3 Papworth

10.3.1 Numbers of patients interviewed and their main characteristics

Seventy-nine patients, 9 of whom were women, were interviewed at assessment. Forty-six patients were suffereing from ischaemic heart disease (IHD), 27 from cardiomyopathy (CM) and 6 had other diagnoses, usually valvular heart disease. The ages of the IHD patients ranged from 28 to 53 with a mean of 44 years; for the CM patients the range was 19 to 50 with a mean age of 36. TABLE 10.1P shows the patients by diagnosis and assessment decision category and TABLE 10.2P gives a breakdown by social class.

The outcome of the 79 patients, following interview at assessment, is shown in TABLE 10.3P. Of the 44 patients who were accepted onto the "definite" waiting list for transplantation, 17 were followed-up in interviews post operatively; of the others, 9 died either before or soon after transplantation, and 15 were either still waiting for their operation or had not reached the 6 month interview date (at 30 April 1984). Of the 17 patients followed-up post operatively it was possible to interview 17 at 6 months, 11 at 1 year and 3 at 2 years. In addition, 21 patients who were transplanted prior to the research commencing, have been interviewed post operatively giving a total of 38 patients interviewed at intervals after their operation, 25 at 6 months, 22 at 1 year, 3 at 18 months, 7 at 2 years and 5 at approximately 30 months, resulting in a total of 62 posttransplant interviews.

10.3.2 Patients at time of assessment

Work situation

In this section of the interview patients were asked specific questions about their working life but were also encouraged to talk about their experiences since they became ill, and about attitudes to any changes in their working life.

A very high proportion, about 89 per cent, of the patients interviewed at assessment were not working and most of these (95%) had given up their job because of their cardiac condition. For the remaining 5 per cent, their illness was a contributing factor to leaving work. Of the 7 patients who were working, only three were subsequently placed on the "definite" waiting list for transplan-

Table 10.1P   Posttransplant follow-up of 79 patients interviewed at assessment (Papworth)

		Numbers		Per Cent
Definitely Accepted			44	55.7%
Interviewed Posttransplantation		17		
—at six months	17			
—at one year	11			
—at two years	3			
Not Interviewed				
Posttransplantation		27		
—transferred to provisional	3			
—died pre transplantation	6			
—died post transplantation	3			
—waiting for transplantation	2			
—received transplant but not yet six months post operation	13			
Provisionally Accepted			14	17.7%
Received Other Cardiac Surgery			10	12.7%
Unsuitable for Surgery			9	11.4%
Died before decision made			2	2.5%
Total			79	100.0%

Table 10.2P   Social class of patients interviewed at assessment (Papworth)

	Numbers by Social Class:					
	I	II	III	IV	V	Total
Manual	0	0	26	11	5	42
Non-Manual	2	15	14	0	0	31
*Total	2	15	40	11	5	73

*Six housewives' social class by husbands' occupation.
       Manual III   4
       Manual IV   2

Table 10.3P   Age/sex by diagnosis for patients interviewed at assessment (Papworth)

Diagnosis	% of sample	Male: Female ratio	Average Age	Age Range
IHD	58.7	10.5:1	44	28–53
CM	34.7	4.4:1	36	19–50
Other	7.6	—	42	32–52
Total	100.0	8: 1	41	19–53

tation. The split between manual and non-manual occupations was 58 per cent manual and 42 per cent non-manual.

Half of the patients interviewed felt that their jobs had been or were being affected by their illness: some had changed to lighter work within their job or had done fewer hours, whereas 11 patients had changed their type of employment completely. TABLE 10.4P gives a breakdown of the length of time the 57 "not working" patients had been away from their jobs. Of those patients not working, 61 per cent would not have a job to return to if they were physically able. Those whose jobs were being held were glad of the financial security and hoped to return eventually to their work.

One of the most frequently expressed comments from those patients not working, was to describe the frustration and anguish caused by their inability to work. A number of reasons were given for this frustration: (i) because they used to enjoy working; (ii) because they missed the social contact of work; (iii) because they felt denied their function in life or (iv) because their families were suffering financially and/or emotionally. Several patients said that it was their working life that they missed most since their illness. Because they were not working their whole normal pattern of life was disrupted. For many of these people the alternative to work was confinement to the house, or perhaps to a hospital bed. Those patients (fewer in number) who said that they had adjusted reasonably well to not working, usually enjoyed interests which helped to keep them busy. Some men had taken over the housekeeping role while their wives went out to work and found some fulfillment therefore in doing something useful.

Table 10.4P   Length of time not working for patients interviewed at assessment (Papworth)

Length of Time	Number of Patients	
	No	Percent
< 6 Months	22	33.8
6–11 Months	15	23.1
1–2 Years	15	23.1
> 2 Years	13	20.0
Total:	65	100.0

The resilience and adaptability of some of the patients with regard to their working life since their illness was very striking. Eleven people interviewed had changed their jobs in an effort to keep working despite their illness. Even so, some of them had to eventually give up on the second physically less-demanding occupation.

A change of job could mean a loss of self esteem, lack of job satisfaction and perhaps financial constraints. Sometimes resentment at employers' attitudes was expressed. One man commented that in the nine years of his illness his main worry had been holding down a job. If heart disease is mentioned to employers, he commented, they "don't want to know". There was a feeling of being "thrown on the scrapheap" because of an illness. Several patients were particu-

121

larly distressed at the loss of their businesses, while some found it difficult to sit back while others ran them. One man who was still working at the time of interview said that although he was doing his job just as well as before his illness, he felt that he was not being promoted as quickly as would have been possible if he had not been suffering from heart disease.

Of the nine women interviewed at assessment, five were housewives and all said that their ability to look after their home and family had been severely limited by their illness. Their husbands work was usually disrupted in some way. One man had given up his job completely to take care of his wife. Others had had long periods away from work, while some were trying to cope with their job and look after the home.

Everyday activities

After working life, the other important areas of daily activity discussed at interview were: (i) Looking After the Home; (ii) Interests and Hobbies; and (iii) Social life. Patients were asked to list their usual activities under these three headings, and to say to what degree each activity had been affected by their illness. TABLE 10.5P summarizes the extent to which these areas of activities were restricted. In all three areas, over 90 per cent of patients were restricted in some way and on average 50 per cent of patients had given up all activities completely.

(i) Looking After The Home

For both men and women, the usual activities around the home had been affected by their illness. For the men it was most often the gardening, decorating and general repairs which had been the most neglected. Although many of the men were spending a great deal of time at home, they could usually only manage very light chores. Sometimes, even jobs like washing-up and making tea were found to be too much of an effort. Several men commented on how much they resented having to ask a friend or relative to do repair jobs around the house while they looked on helpless. These sorts of comments occurred again and again throughout the assessment interviews. For the women, perhaps especially the housewives, this was the area of daily activity which was most affected by their illness. If they could manage any job around the house it was only very light chores. For them, the inability to look after the home and family was both frustrating and distressing. One woman said she wanted the operation because "then I'll feel like a normal mum and wife and be able to share in life all the things the family do".

(i) *Hobbies and Interests*

The activities under this heading fell into four main categories. The first was sporting interests both playing and watching. A wide variety of sports were mentioned at interview, ranging from squash, badminton, cycling, tennis, football and cricket to fishing, darts and snooker. Sometimes, playing sport had been replaced by watching but often even this had to be replaced by simply viewing sport on television. The second main category was family activities. These included walking, boating, caravaning, country drives or just playing with the

Table 10.5P   Restriction on daily activities of patients interviewed at assessment (Papworth)

Restriction	Looking After Home		Interests/Hobbies		Social Life	
	No.	%	No.	%	No.	%
None	36	46.2	34	43.6	39	50.0
None/Limited	21	26.9	28	35.9	7	9.0
Limited	18	23.1	11	14.1	26	33.3
Same or N/A	3	3.8	5	6.4	6	7.7
*Total	78	100.0	78	100.0	78	100.0

*Note: One Patient in hospital for brief time since becoming ill and could not assess extent of restrictions.

children. For many people, most of their interests apart from work, revolved around outings with the family and these were sorely missed. A third category could be labelled community activities and they ranged from church, social and charity work to committee interests in local organisations like P.T.A. or the British Legion.

All these interests and hobbies had been seriously disrupted by illness, the patients often experiencing feelings of loneliness and social isolation as a result. Attempts were often made to replace usual activities with less active pursuits. People forced to spend most of their time either at home or in hospital tried to allay the inevitable boredom in their daily lives by doing more reading, crosswords and puzzles, watching more television or perhaps taking up a new interest in something like home computing, stamp collecting, model making, CB radio, cooking or knitting. Time and again, however, patients would comment on a loss of concentration since their illness, which made even reading an effort. These patients had reached the stage of spending most of their days "just sitting".

Some patients found it very difficult to adapt to inactivity. One man had spent his whole life involved in outdoor work and interests; he bred Dobermans, kept horses, went shooting, attended country shows and tended his greenhouses. His illness brought all this to a halt. Many patients when asked what they missed most from their life before their illness, said that it was the freedom to get out and do what they wanted to do when they wanted to do it.

(iii) *Social Life*

While a majority of patients questioned about their social life commented simply that it was "non existent", some said that it was limited to the occasional visit to friends or relatives or entertaining a few close friends at home. All the usual aspects of an active social life were seriously affected by illness, ranging from outings to the pub or a restaurant and attending a play or concert to dancing and parties.

Some patients found that their illness applied emotional and psychological, as well as physical, constraints in their social contacts. Large gatherings of people were "not easy" to cope with; other patients could not be "bothered" to see people other than very close friends, or quickly felt tired and irritable in company. Social activities were also restricted by more practical difficulties like not being able to sit still for any length of time, always needing to be close to toilet facilities, relying on others to drive, needing fine weather to go out, and of course financial problems caused by being unable to work. When the effort was made to attend a social outing, everything had to be planned well in advance to ensure enough rest prior to the event, and usually the evening would end in returning home early.

Family Relationships

There can be no doubt that a serious cardiac illness imposes a strain on family relationships. Families may suffer because of the patient's inability to work, not only in terms of financial hardship, but also in terms of the potential bad-temper and irritability of the patient. As he/she is often spending a good deal of time at home, these feelings can be vented on the family. It is not only an inability to work that can cause the patient to be ill-tempered; feeling physically awful produces the same effect as does boredom, restlessness and sheer frustration.

The patients interviewed at assessment had often gone through, or were going through, a phase of feeling a burden to their wife and/or their family. "I find it very difficult to sit back and be waited on by my wife and son". There is often an initial difficulty in adjusting to the new circumstances of having a formerly active husband or wife, suddenly becoming a near invalid. The spouse is often considered by the patient to be over protective and fussy. Watching a loved one endure a heart attack, a stay in intensive care, perhaps surgery is, as one wife said, enough to make anyone over protective. Usually the spouse was considered to be "very understanding" when it came to making allowances for bad temper.

All these feelings and reaction were very common in the discussions with patients but the most frequent comment of all — usually expressed before any other — was how this crisis had drawn patient and spouse/family together, had made them closer and more aware of each other. The strain of a serious illness in the family, caused problems only for a third of the patients interviewed, and even among these, a better understanding and a closer relationship was often the final result. Sometimes this effect came from the realisation of the seriousness of the patient's illness.

Patients often expressed concern about the effect of their illness on relationships with children. Children could take a while to adjust to the new situation at home and to accept dad's new crankiness. It was felt that when they did understand what was happening they could be perhaps less boisterous and argumentative, "less natural", subdued even. Mostly, however, children seem to accept things very quickly and be most supportive.

Attitudes to Illness and Transplantation

For most patients interviewed at assessment, the initial reaction to discovering the serious nature of their illness was one of shock and distress followed by depression and then acceptance. Comments like: "I was shattered when I was told" and "why did it happen to me?" were common. As far as possible, patients had come to terms with the situation while still attempting to retain some form of independence by fighting against the physical restrictions. "You can't give up — once you give up you're dead". One way of coping was to "remember there is always someone worse off than you". Some patients said that their illness had meant a period of reflection which resulted in a greater appreciation of everything in their life which had previously been taken for granted.

For some patients the possibility of receiving a heart transplant had only recently been discussed, and they were still adjusting to the idea. The attitude expressed by the majority of patients, however, was very favourable. They saw transplantation as a "chance for life" and were fully committed to accepting the opportunity if it was offered. Some patients spoke about the risks involved but saw their chances with a transplant as better than their inevitable death in the very near future. A heart transplant was the only alternative because life without one would not be worth living, it would be a future without hope, "waiting to die". Patients looked forward to an improved quality of life after transplantation and this was the main consideration, over and above length of survival.

Patients arriving in Papworth for a period of assessment, varied on how well informed they were about the operation itself and the post-operative possibilities. After talking to the surgeons, nurses, social worker and other patients, they felt much better informed about the risks as well as the chances for a normal life. They were grateful for the frank discussions, which were so often mentioned as a feature of the assessment. They felt relieved, reassured and most of all hopeful for the future.

Quality of Life

When asked about their quality of life since their illness, most patients spoke about how everything in their life had been affected, and how useless they felt and about the constant physical discomfort of their existence. The main physical problems experienced by these patients were breathlessness, pain on exertion, tiredness, loss of appetite, coughing and fluid retention, all of which made even walking a short distance, a great effort. Physical restriction dominated everything, even making sleeping, or lying down in bed very difficult, or for some, impossible. For most patients, the distance they could walk had been reduced to a few yards, ranging from ten to a hundred; some patients could walk further on a good day.

The feeling of frustration patients felt at not being able to do any of their former activities, recurred in discussions of quality of life. Their illness had had a total effect on their normal way of life and they spoke of the things they missed most. These varied for different patients; for some it was work, others it was sports and social life or enjoying the home and family. Some people spoke of the loneliness which was part of being housebound or being in hospital, of how the days dragged and the nights were dreaded. One man said that he used to have such a zest for life and his willpower was always strong, but now he felt frightened. Other patients spoke of "existing, not living", "I'm clinging on to life but nothing is left really". Quality of life was "non-existent", "very poor" or "nil". A patient who was to die a few days after his assessment and interview said, "Recently I haven't been able to do anything. I have felt ill and have been walking a few yards when absolutely necessary. I feel I am getting worse. Quality of life is nil."

Perhaps some of the comments above give the impression that all these patients were completely miserable, albeit with good reason. Surprisingly in general that was not true. Patients often spoke reluctantly, or with a wry smile, about how bad things were. Some derive much comfort from a supportive family and close friends, a religious faith perhaps, or just an inbuilt optimism and determination to survive.

10.3.3. Patients posttransplant

Thirty-eight patients were interviewed at intervals after their transplant operation. Twenty-five were seen at six months, 22 at one year, three between one and two years, seven at two years and five between two and three years, giving a total of 62 interviews.

Patients were questioned regarding return to normal activity in the areas of working life, of looking after the home and of social life. They were asked also about their attitude to transplantation and their quality of life since the operation. Thus these interviews were able to explore further our observations (reported in Chapter Nine using scores from Section II of the NHP) that posttransplant far fewer patients felt that their health was causing problems with aspects of their lives. Table 10.5P shows the extent of restriction on daily activity. Most patients suffered very little restriction and were able to pursue more of their usual activities and to pursue them more frequently than pretransplant. For some patients usual activities were combined with new interests, and for others there were still restrictions in some areas.

Working Life

Of the 38 patients interviewed, 4 were full-time housewives and mothers. Of the remaining 34 patients, 19 (56%) returned to work, 16 (47%) to full time employment.

Of the 15 patients not working, one has been doing casual work and another four are very active in fund-raising or voluntary work activities either as a whole time career or to keep busy while looking for paid employment. Of the 12 patients still unemployed, 10 are seeking employment and have applied for several jobs over a period of nine months to two years posttransplantation.

Seven of the 19 patients who returned to work, did so in less than six months following their transplantation; a further, eight in less than one year, one more by one year but three could not get a job for over three years following transplantation. One of the 19 has been made redundant after being back at work for over two years.

Sixteen of the 19 patients were able to return to their usual occupation, either because their jobs had been held open or because they were able to obtain employment in the same field. The split between those who had manual and non-manual occupations was 32 per cent and 68 per cent respectively.

The patients returning to work all spoke of feeling quite capable of holding down a full time and sometimes a physically demanding job. Some examples of the manual occupations held by these patients were master baker, taxi driver and milkman. Non-manual occupations included news editing, banking, systems analysis, and sales. Some patients reported working between 50 and 80 hours a week. Two patients working as sales representatives and another two patients "working" as fund raisers (from the 15 patients without paid employment) reported several hundred miles of driving every week, while another patient spent two hours travelling to and from work every day. One patient doing manual work said that he felt tired every few months but coped with this by taking a week off work, returning refreshed. Some patients had eased back into normal employment by spending the first month or so working part time. Patients were questioned about changing to lighter work or shorter hours, but surprisingly few felt this was necessary. Several patients commented that they felt they were doing their job better than during the months/years of illness before transplantation. As well as a return to physical fitness for work, patients report better concentration, and a more relaxed attitude, quicker reactions and improved mental alertness.

About 40 per cent of the employers of those patients who had returned to work had been very supportive from the beginning of the illness, keeping the job open and accepting a gradual return to work, plus the occasional absences for checkups in hospital. Three patients had their own business so they were able to return gradually to an active role plus enjoying the freedom of arranging their own working hours. The remaining patients had been fortunate enough to find new employers who accepted these situations.

Most patients returning to an active working life, found that after a short time their colleagues stopped cosseting them and accepted that they could do their job, working usual hours, without ill effect.

The patients who were not working when interviewed, fell into three main categories. There were those who had really just begun to think about returning to work. During the few months since their transplant they had been quite happy to concentrate on getting fit and enjoying being home with their families. Then there were those who had found alternative interests to their previous work, who were financially secure and therefore did not have to go back to work to earn money. They were just taking their time, keeping their options open and enjoying their interests.

The third category of patients were those who had been looking for work without any success for perhaps several years. Many of them had attended rehabilitation courses where they had been assessed for and advised about suitable employment. These courses usually ran for several weeks and patients had enjoyed being back in a working routine. Not being able to find employment was often distressing, annoying and frustrating, especially as these patients felt perfectly capable of doing a full time job. Sometimes patients were resentful about prospective employers' attitudes. They commented that it was difficult to convince employers that a heart transplant patient can do a normal day's work. Persuading employers to make allowances for the time away from work for checkups was another major hurdle; and then of course there were the complicated problems of insurance and pension schemes, ie passing the medical when opinions between examiners vary as to the classification of transplantation. Some patients, however, believed that the present levels of unemployment were the main obstacle to their getting work, especially in industry.

Some of these patients were facing serious financial problems because of not working, while others spoke of the psychological effects of unemployment, like feeling useless and inferior. Each patient found his own way of keeping busy: some turned to voluntary work like doing decorating jobs for old people, or electrical repairs for neighbours; others ran the home while their wives worked and took up new hobbies, while others again tried to find casual work which would bring in some money. What they all had in common was the determination to find work eventually. One patient recently returned to work nearly four years after receiving his transplant during which time he said he had applied for hundreds of jobs. Other patients commented that their lives were completely normal again, apart from not working.

Looking after the home

Most of the men interviewed post-operatively were able to do the usual jobs around the house that had been neglected during their illness: D.I.Y. and repair work, decorating, shopping and cooking, were all mentioned. Some male patients who were not working had taken on the housekeeping role while their wives went out to work. To some patients, one of the greatest things about being physically fit again, was being able to do jobs around the house which, during their illness, had been done by relatives or friends.

The housewives who were interviewed spoke of the pleasure and relief of being able to look after their home and families once more. In the early months after the operation, some women said they were still restricted with the heavier chores like cleaning windows, and were still working at a slower pace than normal, but they could feel themselves improving every day. One woman at six months post-operatively, said she could now manage quite heavy chores and could shop in town for two or three hours or be on her feet in the kitchen all day, without feeling unduly tired. The husband of one female patient remarked that on returning home from hospital, his wife had spring cleaned the house twice, just for the pleasure of being able to do it after many years of illness before her transplant!

Interests and Hobbies

The range of interests pursued by post-operation transplant patients was impressive. Just about every sport imaginable was mentioned; walking, cycling, swimming and golf were four of the favourites but tennis, badminton, squash and football were also quite commonplace. One patient had enjoyed a skiing holiday a few months before his twelve month interview. Some of these active pastimes had been enjoyed before the patient's illness but several had been taken up as new interests, since receiving the transplant, possibly as a result of trying them out at the "transplant games" but usually because of a desire to maintain and improve their physical fitness. Several patients had embarked on an exercise programme in a local gymnasium to help restore strength to the legs, weakened by inactivity during the long illness. This attitude could result in a patient feeling fitter in himself after his transplant than before his illness, when he had perhaps led a rather sedentary life style.

Some patients reported their participation in these very active hobbies at less than six months after transplantation, while others said that it was between six and twelve months that they really felt well enough to go back out on the golf course, or whatever, although some patients remarked that it was the bad weather which had stopped them "having a go", rather than physical restriction — the summer months were obviously the best time to embark on outdoor activities. The less active sporting interests mentioned included: fishing, shooting, bowling, playing snooker or pool, watching cricket and "messing-about in boats". Another popular type of activity which people were glad to resume was

128

driving and maintaining a car or motorcycle. Enjoying a day out with the family was something which many patients remarked on as being one of the greatest delights of feeling well again.

After transplantation people found that they could enjoy their leisure time at home again. They could now concentrate on reading, drawing, writing, doing crosswords, knitting or just listening to music or watching T.V. Other patients talked of interest in home computing and electronics, model making and carpentry and studying for examinations.

An interest in voluntary work with handicapped or old people, plus various church and other community activities were either resumed or initiated in the months following transplantation. For those people for whom this kind of interest was new, some of them took it up because they could not find paid employment and wanted to keep busy and be useful, others became interested because of a sense of gratitude to society for their medical care and the chance of a new life. Another outlet for this need to "put something back" was involvement in fund raising activities like organising shows, concerts and fetes and attending, perhaps competing in, sponsored sporting events. One patient has spent most of his time since receiving his transplant travelling hundreds of miles a week to attend fund raising activities, give after dinner speeches, open fetes, and visit potential heart transplant patients.

Social Life

Very soon after leaving hospital most patients found very few restrictions to their social life. The activities mentioned included visiting friends, entertaining at home, outings to a pub or restaurant, attending the theatre or concerts and going to dances and parties. Some people remarked that it was marvellous to be able to enjoy a social life again, to be able to stay out late without worrying about feeling unduly tired, and to be meeting up again with friends they haven't seen for months or years. One patient said that for years before his illness, he had led a very busy working life and had been reluctant to go out in the evening. Now he enjoys going out regularly and does not feel tired even though he is working just as hard during the day.

A few patients, however, did talk about a preference for socialising with a small group of close friends particularly in the few months after leaving hospital. They found the larger social gatherings less relaxing. As one patient said, to spend a whole evening recounting recent medical history and perhaps having to deal with rather silly questions about transplantation, could become tedious. Patients ability to cope with larger social groups seemed to improve over time. It also seems to be true that as the idea of cardiac transplantation is more accepted, and the event more commonplace, this kind of problem would appear to be diminishing. The pressure from both the public and the press on a heart transplant patient in 1984 is, generally speaking, a good deal less than it was in 1980.

Home Relationships

One of the main factors which could affect home relationships was the family's response to the return home of a fit and well husband or wife, son or daughter, who had only recently been an invalid, who needed everything done for him/her. It was sometimes very difficult to adjust suddenly to having a normal member of the family around again, particularly if the illness had been a long one. This could cause real problems but mostly things were worked out in time. One patient said he had been impossible to live with when he first went home. He had wanted to do everything immediately and his family still treated him as an invalid, which made him irritable. So they all sat down together and talked it out.

Patients often talked of the pressures placed on their spouse by the illness and operation. The strain and anxiety sometimes created problems, made worse sometimes by the financial constraint resulting from unemployment.

Most patients said that family relationships had improved tremendously since the operation. During their illness they had been so difficult to live with and felt such a burden on their family. "I was becoming a bad tempered old man" said one patient. People spoke of a new closeness in family relations, especially between husband and wife, as a result of all they had been through together. They seemed to be making the most of their life together, appreciating each other's company more and spending more time with each other and sharing things, especially if the patient was not working.

Follow-up care at transplant centre

Patients were asked how they felt about returning to Papworth for their day visits, biopsies and the annual checkup which usually entails a couple of days stay in hospital. They were also asked about the practical aspects of travelling to Papworth from all different parts of the country; getting time off work, coping with a long or difficult journey, and financing the visits.

Visits to the transplant centre become less frequent as time passes, changing from a visit every week just after the operation, to once a month and then to every few months. The majority of patients were glad to reach the last of these stages but most of them said they realised how important it was to be monitored regularly. They were thankful for their transplant and thought that the regular journeys to Papworth were a "small price to pay" for the quality of care and reassurance these visits provided. One patient described it as "a good early warning system". Others said that they felt so well and were leading such normal lives that it was difficult sometimes to accept the constant monitoring, not of an illness, but of health.

Some patients enjoyed the chance for a day out, particularly those with no fixed work commitment who perhaps live within a couple of hours drive of the hospital. They looked forward to meeting up with the other patients, seeing the staff and generally keeping in touch. No one spoke of actually enjoying the cardiac biopsies and the annual investigations of course, but several patients agreed that thinking about them beforehand was worse than the real thing. It was difficult not to worry a little about what they may reveal. As one patient said, "the possibility that they will find something, is always at the back of your mind". Another commented that he didn't look forward to the results of the test because really he didn't want to know.

For some patients the journey to Papworth, from Scotland or the West Country for example, was difficult, tiring and expensive. These were the people especially relieved when the visits became less frequent but they still thought the effort well worthwhile. Where the train connections were really a problem, patients would need to stay overnight in "bed and breakfast" accommodation in the village, but, as one patient said, this was a better alternative to rushing about trying to do the journey in one day. Another patient described the journey as an "unavoidable irritation". Several patients said they preferred not to have to make the journey because they would rather be at work or at home, but they didn't see any point in moaning about it. A cheerful uncomplaining attitude was much better. There was praise for local hospitals and their staff but most people said they would prefer to hear the OK from Papworth. Most of the patients who were working found their employers were reasonable about taking time off for checkups.

Disadvantages of the operation

When asked about any disadvantages of the transplant operation, most patients reply was they didn't know of any. They spoke of how little they could do before the operation and how much they could do now. The minor health problems, which were usually side effects of the drugs that they were taking, plus the difficulty for some people finding a job since their transplant, were not seen as disadvantages as such; rather as irritating complications which meant that their lives were not completely back to how they were before their illness.

Some drugs taken after transplantation, usually in decreasing doses over the years, can cause extra hair growth and produce a Cushingoid appearance. Several patients suffered from these problems but found them acceptable. A more worrying problem for some patients was the weight gain which subsequently they found very difficult to shed. Other fairly distressing complaints were acne, skin rashes and warts on the hand, all of which could be rather persistent. Temporary problems in the months immediately following the operation included muscle weakness in arms and legs, hand cramp, perhaps slight oedema or breathlessness and some pain in the chest where the ribs were mending. These were all, of course, minor health problems compared with those suffered before transplantation. The only problem which seemed to get people down however was the weight gain and their inability to lose this extra weight even though they were keeping to the recommended low-fat diet.

Something else which patients had to learn to live with, was the uncertainty of length of survival. Thinking and planning for the future, especially when you have a young family, is difficult when you really don't know how long you'll be around. Several patients said they dealt with this by concentration on the quality of life rather than speculating on length of life.

Attitudes to transplantation

When asked whether transplantation had been worthwhile for them, all patients said that it had; even those who had experienced a very difficult recovery period in hospital after the operation, or were still having problems with infection or rejection episodes several years on. Some people said that they had always believed in cardiac transplantation and had been confident that they would survive. Other patients were a little surprised that everything had gone so well that they had made such steady progress and were getting better all the time. Many patients said that it had been a great success for them and that they would recommend it to anyone else who was offered the chance. It was the quality of life that was spoken of most — the nearness to normality which was "like being re-born" after such a debilitating illness. Another common remark was, "if it all ended tomorrow it would still have been worthwhile".

A few patients spoke of the responsibility transplantation brings to the way you take care of yourself and generally conduct your life. Not just for your own sake and your family's but for people who may benefit from the programme in the future. A good yardstick was to try never to do anything which would cause any upset to the donor's next of kin or to the surgical/nursing team at Papworth, or indeed to the tax payers.

Quality of life

In discussing quality of life posttransplant, the accent was on the contrast to life shortly before the operation. The lack of restrictions, especially at the interview one year after transplantation were, to these patients, remarkable after the confinement of the serious illness. Most people said they were completely back to normal and were leading a full and active life, doing exactly what they wanted to do, and feeling happy and content. Some patients said that it was not until their health was restored that they could appreciate how ill they had been. Regained independence in looking after the home, in driving and walking, in personal hygiene even, was very satisfying. Freedom from unpleasant symptoms, like breathlessness, chest pains, tiredness and oedema, added greatly to quality of life. Those patients that had been ill for several years, some of them for most of their lives, perhaps particularly appreciated the difference.

A few patients felt that their quality of life would not be completely restored until they could find some work. This was especially true for the men who had been trying to find employment for a long time, sometimes years. As one patient said, "if I could get a little job, life would be complete". Some patients felt that their physical condition was not quite as good as before their illness. Sometimes this was temporary as with something like muscle weakness, but for others it was longer lasting, like weight gain for instance.

Whereas before the operation, the patients rated their quality of life, on a scale of 0 to 10, somewhere between 0 and 4; posttransplant the scores range from 8 to 10 plus. There were some patients who said that their quality of life was higher than it had been before their illness. They were not just back to normal, they felt better, were even more active, physically and mentally fitter and more content. People talked about, "living life to the full", "making up lost time", seeing life from a different angle, not taking the good things in life for granted anymore, a feeling of being in extra time — "every day is a bonus". One patient said he had gained, "two good years I would not have had for transplant". Patients talked about the fact that they were more aware of their physical condition now, than before their illness, and had perhaps taken up sports they played in their youth or developed new activities, in a determination to hold onto their new fitness, and their new life. The patients with young families were particularly glad of the opportunity to enjoy their children growing up; not just surviving to watch them growing, but having the quality of life which enabled them to share in their activities to the full.

A few patients, usually people who had worked very hard at their job and perhaps had not had a great deal of time for outside interests, including family, commented that their priorities had altered since their transplant. They were working hard, but also trying to have time for a fuller family and social life, and a physical fitness programme. One patient said that he had a much calmer outlook since his transplant. Little things that used to upset him didn't seem important after what he and his family had been through.

In summary, the general opinion was that cardiac transplantation brought bonus years in terms of survival, but most important, with the majority, a rich quality of life.

10.4 Summary

Our second approach to the assessment of the quality of life of patients, both before and after transplant, was to conduct semi-structured interviews with open-ended questions. We collected information on working life; everyday activities; hobbies; social life; family relationships; patients' attitudes to their illness and to transplantation, plus views as to their quality of life.

In total 277 interviews were held involving patients at assessment and after operation at six months, twelve months and two years. Although these were conducted separately by a different interviewer at each centre, the impressions that emerge are strikingly similar.

Before operation patients spoke of depression, frustration, feelings of degradation, immobility and uselessness. Though some were apprehensive, they were most anxious to receive a transplant. Six months posttransplant they used adjectives such as tremendous, fantastic and magic when describing how they felt. At one year more than half the surviving patients had returned to work; almost all were enjoying a broad range of leisure interests, including fund raising and voluntary work. They gave evidence of a remarkably unrestricted lifestyle after transplant and a near normal quality of life.

11. Comments on the Epidemiology of Heart Transplantation

11.1 Relative frequency with which conditions have been referred and treated to date

Cases treated by heart transplantation have fallen into the following groups: ischaemic heart disease (ICD 410-414), certain cardiomyopathies particularly dilated cardiomyopathy (included in ICD 425), and valvular heart disease (only the acquired form of which is distinguished as ICD 394-396). In the two centres combined, the ratios of these diagnoses amongst patients who received transplants during 1982–1984 were 10:6:1. As was shown in TABLE 2.7 this average conceals a somewhat higher proportion or cardiomyopathies amongst the patients at Papworth (41 per cent of the total as compared with 31 per cent at Harefield). Very similar ratios exists amongst the totals of patients referred and assessed.

11.2 Trends in mortality rates for these conditions

No morbidity data are routinely available for studying and epidemiology of the potential demand for the operation. A prognosis of imminent death is one of the most important criteria for heart transplantation, so cause-specific mortality data are not inappropriate for the purpose, although the data they yield can only be regarded as rough approximations. Published mortality data for England and Wales, with their combined population of just under 50 million in 1982, are available in a suitable form for this purpose. For Scotland however, with a population in the same year of just over 5 million suitably disaggregated data are not readily available. The major part of this Chapter is therefore concerned with England and Wales; Scotland is considered in Section 11.5.

As a total health problem ischaemic heart disease which caused 4,400 deaths in England and Wales in persons under 50 years of age in 1982 greatly outweighs the importance of cardiomyopathy and acquired valvular heart disease. In the same age group in the same year, all of the cardiomyopathies (the sub-groups are not distinguished in routinely published mortality data) caused 195 deaths, and acquired valvular disease of the heart 116. Of these the numbers under the age of 15 years were 5, 49 and 3 respectively.

The long standing rise in death *rates* from ischaemic heart disease discontinued about ten years ago. Age specific mortality analyses show the following details:

Ischaemic heart disease (FIGURE 11.1)

— Between 1967 and 1973, rates increased in both sexes for age groups 45-64 and 65-74, increases being slightly greater in the middle-aged groups;
— Over the same period there was no change in rate for either sex in people aged 25-44 years;

Figure 11.1: Trends in age specific death rates from ischaemic heart disease (410-414) England and Wales

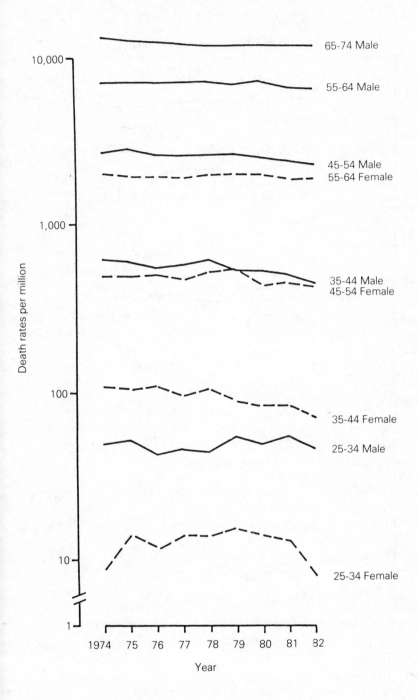

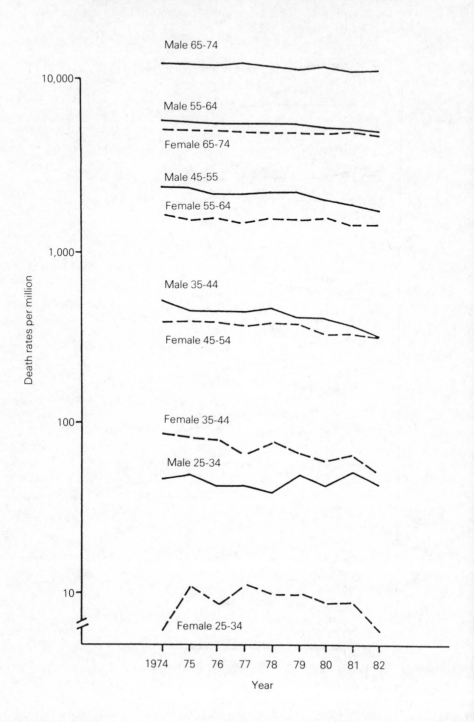

Figure 11.2: Trends in age specific death rates from acute myocardial infarction (410) England and Wales

Male 65-74

Male 55-64

Female 65-74

Male 45-55

Female 55-64

Male 35-44

Female 45-54

Female 35-44

Male 25-34

Female 25-34

Death rates per million

1974 75 76 77 78 79 80 81 82

Year

— Between 1974 and 1982 there were decreases in rate, which were sharper than the previous increases, for both sexes in age groups 35-44 and 45-54 years;

— There was no consistent change in rate in age groups 25-34 years. In group 65-74 years, both sexes showed a slight fall.

Acute Myocardial Infarction (FIGURE 11.2)

— With the exception of age group 25-34 years, which showed no change, both sexes in all groups showed declines in *rates* which are sharper than those shown for the same age groups for ischaemic heart disease. (Acute myocardial infarction accounts for about 72 per cent of all mortality attributed to ischaemic heart disease.)

11.3 Numbers of persons dying from these conditions

In many respects the *crude* numbers of people in need of health care suffering from disease are more useful statistics for planning than are rates. The numbers of people aged 15-49 years dying from the three conditions in England and Wales in 1982 (IHD 4,400, cardiomyopathy 195 and acquired valvular disease 116) give ratios of 37.9 : 1.7 : 1. Thus comparison with the ratios for patients transplanted (restated in Section 11.1) shows that at the present time although cardiomyopathy and valvular disease of the heart cause fewer deaths, heart transplantation is more important in the treatment of those suffering from them relative to the frequency of deaths from these diseases, than it is in the treatment of ischaemic heart disease.

The *number* of deaths from ischaemic heart disease in persons aged under 65 years has also, as might be expected from trends in rates, decreased since 1973 (FIGURE 11.3). Overall by 1982 about 5,000 fewer deaths were reported (a 13 per cent fall over ten years). Deaths from acquired valvular disease have fallen too (the number over the same period being 440, an 80 per cent fall) (FIGURE 11.4.) (This fall has been exaggerated by a change in the International Classification of Disease; by the criteria set out in the eighth revision it would probably have been about 40 per cent.) In contrast the number of deaths certified as being due to cardiomyopathy has risen sharply from 133 in 1974 to 391 in 1982 (FIGURE 11.5). This does not necessarily mean that the disease is becoming commoner; to an unknown extent it may reflect an improved ability to distinguish cardiomyopathy from myocardial ischaemia of arterial origin. Presumably many, though not all, of the 195 decedents were candidates for heart transplantation. It is an informed opinion (Goodwin [1984]) that in the group 15-49 years, between 50 per cent and 60 per cent of cases suffering from cardiomyopathy could have been helped by transplantation. The rise in reported death rates from cardiomyopathy is evident in most age/sex groups (FIGURE 11.6); the extent to which this is attributable to changing diagnostic practice is not known.

It is reasonable for present purposes to assume that persons certified as dying of acute myocardiac infarction either die suddenly, or so rapidly that they are not considered for cardiac transplantation. Thus potential candidates for the operation are those who died of IHD but did not have AMI (ICD Categories 411-414). In 1982, therefore, there was a maximum of 1,228 IHD deaths *under 50* in persons who might potentially have been seriously considered for transplantation (TABLE 11.7); the *actual* number of potential candidates is unknown

Figure 11.3 : Trends in number of deaths from ischaemic heart disease (410-414) England and Wales (persons under 65)

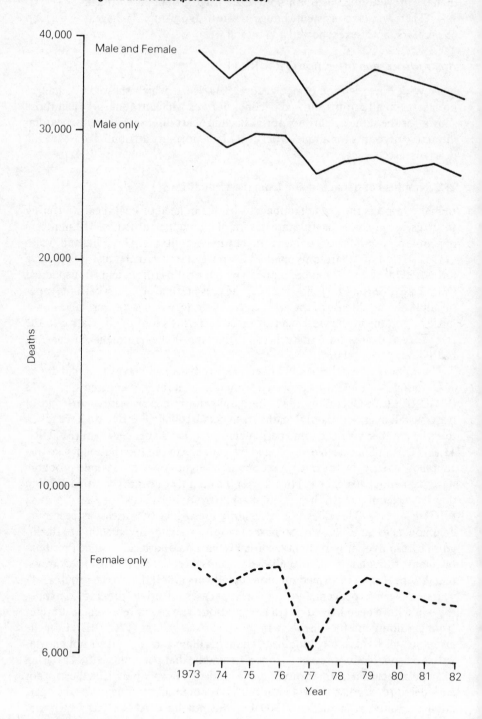

Figure 11.4: Trends in number of deaths from acquired disease of the heart valves (394-395) England and Wales (persons under 65)

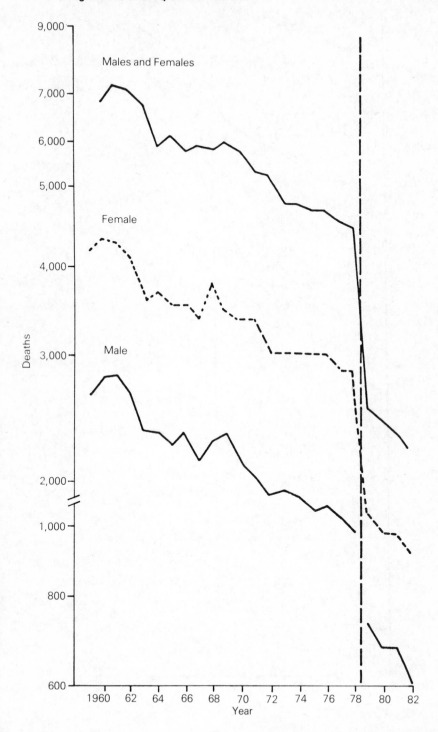

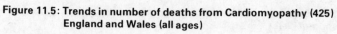
Figure 11.5: Trends in number of deaths from Cardiomyopathy (425) England and Wales (all ages)

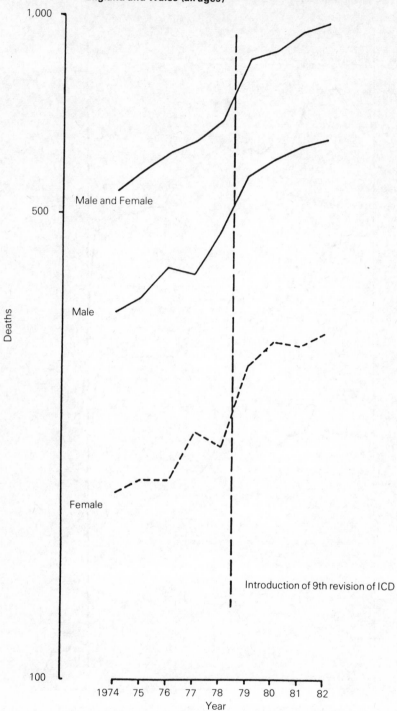

Male and Female

Male

Female

Introduction of 9th revision of ICD

Deaths

1,000

500

100

Year

1974 75 76 77 78 79 80 81 82

**Figure 11.6: Trends in age specific death rates from Cardiomyopathy (425)
England and Wales**

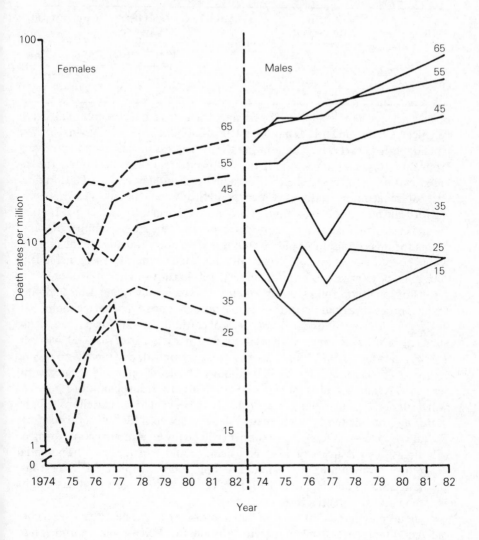

Table 11.7   Gross deaths from Ischaemic heart disease in England and Wales in certain age groups in 1980 and 1982

	All IHD (410–414)		AMI (410)		Other IHD (411–414)		Cardiomyopathy (425)	
	1980	1982	1980	1982	1980	1982	1980	1982
Ages 15–49	4932	4400	3699	3172	1223	1228	175	195
50–64 years	30301	28742	22544	21106	7757	7637	295	316

however. It could be established by tracing case notes from a sample of all death certificates coded under ICD numbers 410-414. If all 1,228 cases had in fact been candidates for heart transplantation; if the present rate of fall in numbers dying from this cause continues, and if the death rate represents accurately the incidence of potential cases, then in a decade there would be about 1,000 terminal cases of ischaemic heart disease which theoretically could be considered as suitable for transplantation. This figure is no more than an informed guess. If every second case in this age group is considered suitable, the annual number of transplants for this condition would be 500; if it were every fourth case the number would be 250. The factors which will influence what actually happens include the suitability of alternative forms of surgery; this in turn will be influenced by the results of long term follow-up of patients who have undergone transplant and by-pass procedures and the unforeseeable influence of advancing technology.

Very crude projections of suitable cases of cardiomyopathy can be made using similarly broad reasoning. All deaths reported in this group of disease have risen 1.6 fold over ten years. If this rate of increase continued, and there is no way of knowing whether it will, there will be about 1,500 deaths in this ICD category in ten years. Again, not all of these will be candidates for transplantation. Only 320 will be under 50, and in this group probably 40 per cent to 50 per cent will not be suffering from dilated cardiomyopathy, leaving between 130 and 160 who are; if the rate of increase is less, these numbers will be fewer. Among people dying of this disease also, a survey of death certificates could help to clarify the potential scope for transplantation. If it should become common practice to offer transplants to infants and children the influence this will have on numbers can be ignored because potential cases are so few.

Such a small number of cases of valvular disease of the heart have been considered suitable for transplantation to date, and the decrease in its mortality is so rapid, that this condition is not likely to be an important factor in projections.

In summary, we can make estimates of extremes by adding maximum to maximum and minimum to minimum. Thus it can be argued that the number of cases which may be considered suitable for cardiac transplantation aged *under* 50 years in the early 1990's in England and Wales will not exceed 1,200 per annum, or be less than 380 per annum; 790 is midway between the extremes. However, as the upper age limit is raised over 50, as is already the case at Harefield, less restrictive age criteria bring with them a large increase in numbers for each additional year of age. In 1982 there were six times as many deaths between the age of 50 and 64 for the two diagnostic groups combined as there were between 15 and 49 (TABLE 11.7). Numbers will also be influenced by "repeat" transplants and by changes in the proportion of cardiologists willing to refer patients.

These figures of course relate to possible future "demand" without attempting to relate it to the costs and benefits, or the likely level of provision.

11.4 Geographical variation in mortality from ischaemic heart disease and cardiovascular surgery

Age adjusted mortality rates from the two ICD categories for coronary artery disease vary considerably from region to region, and are generally highest in the north and west of the country and lowest in the south and east (TABLE 11.8). There are too few deaths from cardiomyopathy or valvular disease to permit a meaningful regional analysis of rates.

There are two sources of information about the distribution of operations on the heart and the intrathoracic vessels in England and Wales. One is the Hospital Inpatient Enquiry (HIPE) which has been running for over thirty years (Office of Population Censuses and Surveys [1984]) and the other a special cardiac surgical register (CSR) (English [1978]; English et al [1984]). There are important differences between the two. CSR sets out to keep a register of all cardiac surgical operations in the country and depends for its information on the submission of standard returns to the Society of Cardiac Surgeons by the responsible surgeons; on the other hand HIPE depends in general upon the routine processing of the routine case records of a representative 10 per cent sample of all discharges. As regards geographical analyses, whereas CSR's recent report classifies geographical distribution by location of hospital, HIPE publications classify by permanent residence of patients. Finally, HIPE publishes its results for each year annually, but the recently published CSR figures are means for a six-year period.

Table 11.8   Standardised mortality ratios for Ischaemic heart disease and Acute Myocardial Infarction for Wales and English Regional Health Authorities

	IHD (410–414)				AMI (410)			
	Male		Female		Male		Female	
	1980	1981	1980	1981	1980	1981	1980	1981
Northern	115	115	121	124	117	120	126	132
Yorkshire	111	114	114	121	114	117	115	121
Trent	102	103	105	103	99	100	106	99
East Anglian	84	88	91	91	80	76	86	86
North West Thames	87	89	84	89	83	87	83	87
North East Thames	89	92	87	87	91	92	89	89
South East Thames	91	91	87	87	94	93	90	87
South West Thames	88	88	88	86	86	84	87	81
Wessex	98	91	93	92	99	88	90	90
Oxford	88	88	92	90	83	85	87	88
South Western	96	93	93	90	107	104	107	97
West Midlands	99	100	101	100	90	92	91	91
Mersey	105	107	105	107	108	109	111	113
North Western	115	119	118	119	124	129	125	125
Wales	108	113	106	106	106	109	106	107

These differences in method however do not explain wholly the differences in reported surgery rates. On the one hand grossing up the HIPE sample gives a number of about 27,000 operations performed in England and Wales in 1980.

143

For 1982, the HIPE estimate had risen to over 33,000 for England alone. On the other hand, the mean annual figure, for the United Kingdom including Scotland and Northern Ireland, recorded for the six years 1977−1982 by CSR was only 14,000. Different definitions of cardiac operations are responsible for a major element of the discrepancies in these estimates: the HIPE data, unlike the CSR, include catheterisations. But TABLE 11.9, comparing the regional rates for cardiac surgery per 10,000 population by quoting the CSR means for the period 1977−1982 and the equivalent means from HIPE data, shows that not only are there large absolute differences between the two data sets, but nor is there a consistent relationship between them. Without a detailed reconciliation of these two sets of data to explain the differences, no geographical analysis can be interpreted with confidence.

11.5 Scotland

In Scotland in 1982 between the ages of *25 and 54 years* 3302 men and 1178 women a total of 4480 died of ischaemic heart disease (ICD 410-414); available data do not specify numbers aged 15 to 49, nor do they distinguish those dying from either acute myocardial infarction or from the cardiomyopathies (SHHD [1984]). FIGURE 11.10 shows that over the past decade, age specific rates for each sex have been rather higher than in England and Wales, and have remained constant or tended slowly to fall — with the exception of men aged 35-44 and 45-54 among whom the fall has been 20 per cent to 30 per cent.

Table 11.9   Comparison of estimates of cardiac operations from the hospital inpatient enquiry and the cardiac surgery register: rates per 10,000 population for England by Regional Health Authority

Regional Health Authority	HIPE Mean 1977−1982	Cardiac Surgery Register Mean 1977−1982
Northern	5.1	1.9
Yorkshire	5.2	2.0
Trent	5.9	1.6
East Anglia	4.5	1.8
N W Thames	5.6	4.3
N E Thames	5.7	3.6
S E Thames	7.4	4.1
S W Thames	5.6	2.1
Wessex	5.9	1.7
Oxford	5.6	0.8
South Western	3.4	0.8
West Midlands	5.1	1.7
Mersey	4.1	2.2
North Western	5.8	3.8

The population in Scotland aged 15-49 in 1982 was in the order of 2.4 million compared with just under 24 million in the same age group in the same year in England and Wales. Even though, as we have seen the mortality rates for IHD in Scotland are a little higher than England and Wales, and the rate of fall a little lower, an estimate of a demand from 80 cases of IHD and 15 of cardiomyopathy in a population one tenth of the size in 1994 is in line with the arguments set out above.

11.6 Comparison between our estimates and the demand projections of the British Cardiac Society

The projections in this chapter have been made independently from those in a report from the Council of the British Cardiac Society of November 1983 (British Cardiac Society [1984]). Nevertheless, even though the methods used in the two approaches are quite different, the estimates derived are broadly similar.

Estimates in the report of the British Cardiac Society were based on a canvass of nine cardiac centres, Brighton, Chertsey, Edinburgh, Glasgow, Hammersmith, Hillingdon, Newcastle, Nottingham and Southampton, each of which was asked to predict the number of cases, under the age of 50, of dilated cardiomyopathy and of irremediable ischaemic cardiac failure, which might be suitable for transplantation in the forthcoming year. To this were added 30 cases of hypertrophic cardiomyopathy and 50 cases of otherwise inoperable congenital heart disease, giving a total of 750 cases per year. This approach depends upon an estimate of what an epidemiologist uses as the numerator of his incidence rate, and its is classified in very precise terms. The catchment area of none of the collaborating centres can be clearly defined however; thus, although it is assumed that the national yield is based on the national population, no more and no less, there is no way of being sure of this. The referral patterns may involve duplication under some circumstances, and under other, there may be parts of the population from which there is a misleadingly low referral rate.

In contrast the approach employed in this report uses as a starting point a precise and clearly defined denominator, namely the annual estimates made by the O.P.C.S. of the total population of England and Wales, and then considers the causes of death yielded by this in a year. The classification of cause of death is inaccurate, as we have pointed out for instance in the distinction between some cases of ischaemic heart disease and cardiomyopathy; moreover it provides no information about the suitability of the case of any decedent, in the terminal states of the illness, for cardiac transplantation.

Taking these differences into account, for England and Wales the estimate of 750 cases under 50 years of age in 1984 from the British Cadiac Society compares remarkably closely with our median figure of 790 in the same age group in 1994. Allowing 100 for Scotland, a round figure of 900 can therefore, it seems, be reasonably taken as a basis for planning in the under 50 age group over the next ten years. Increasing the age at which surgery is performed will of course greatly increase the numbers of potential candidates.

11.7 Summary

The principal indications for cardiac transplantation are dilated cardiomyopathy and ischaemic heart disease. Although reported mortality from the former is on the increase and from the latter on the decrease, the prevalence of terminal ischaemic heart disease is so much greater than that of dilated cardiomyopathy that changes in demand for cardiac transplantation over the next decade can be expected to be influenced more by its suitability for treating the latter, than by any other biological factor. This is especially relevant to people aged over fifty years. A professional factor which may change is the widely differing attitude of cardiologists about the appropriateness of the operation.

Although the prevalence of ischaemic heart disease increases with age, it does

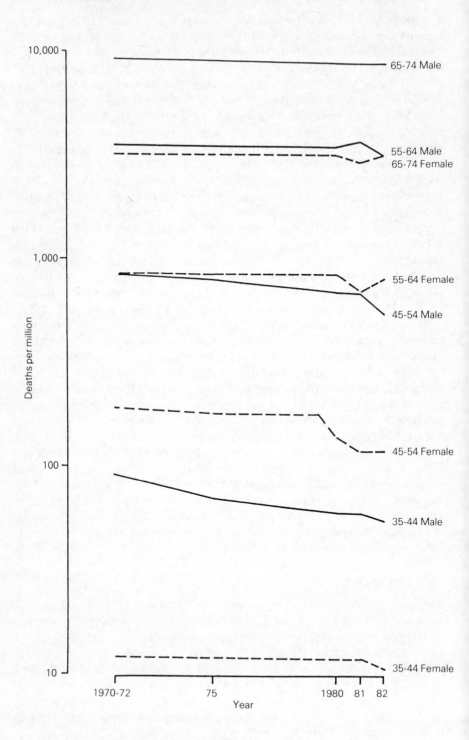

Figure 11.10: Trends in age specific death rates from ischaemic heart disease (410-414) Scotland

not necessarily follow that the prevalence of suitable cases increases at the same rate; presumably older patients will have contra-indications to transplantation because of other disease.

On the basis of a series of simple, but unconfirmable assumptions, it can be argued that the annual demand (in England and Wales) in ten years which will be made by people *under fifty years of age* may in round figures be between 380 and 1200 per year — the median of these is 790. Allowing for 100 from Scotland a very approximate round figure of the order of 900 is reached for that age group.

It is not possible to estimate this number more accurately from published data and we would therefore recommend that a full epidemiological investigation be undertaken to determine how present demand for the operation relates to potential national demand. This would probably best be done by analysis of case records identified though a probability sample of death certificates.

There are large of unsystematic discrepancies between HIPE and CSR data on regional rates of cardiac surgery. We would recommend that the two main data colletion bodies undertake a full reconciliation of these data sets, and then that the relevant referral practice and patterns be investigated further to clarify the policy implications of these existing regional varitions in cardiac surgery for the planning of transplantation services.

12. Comparative Costs and Benefits

12.1 Introduction

In the preceding chapters we have, as far as is possible in the absence of an adequate control group, attempted to measure the additional costs and patient benefits of the heart transplant programmes. Throughout, we have aimed to compare transplantation with "conventional" medical management of such patients. Although such conservative management may be the only alternative therapy for this particular group of patients, there are clearly many other alternative ways in which the scarce resources might be used; perhaps in the treatment of patients with other cardiac disease, or more widely in the provision of therapies to different patient care groups within the NHS.

It is, however, quite beyond the remit of our study to assess the costs and benefits of the many and varied services which may be seen as competing for a share of the limited pool of resources. Ideally, policy makers should have, and perhaps eventually will have, a folio of studies providing comparable estimates of the costs and benefits of the majority of health care interventions.

Currently, because the methods used in estimating costs and measuring benefits are still being refined, any comparisons between separate evaluations of different treatments must be made with extreme caution. To assist such comparisons, we have collected data on a number of coronary artery bypass graft (CABG) operations at each centre. Costs have been estimated using the same costing conventions and methods as those used for the transplant patients. Similarly, patient benefits have been assessed using the Nottingham Health Profile (NHP).

It must be stressed that we provide such estimates for CABG patients *not* because the relevant treatment choice should be between transplantation and bypass grafting, nor to attempt an evaluation of CABG, but rather to provide specific cost and benefit "benchmarks" against which our measurement for transplant patients can be "calibrated".

12.2 Costs of coronary artery bypass graft patients: Operation to discharge

We focussed simply on the costs of coronary artery bypass grafting in the period from the operation to discharge. Our reasons were twofold. First it reflects the need to address a question commonly posed to us as to the comparison of costs for CABG patients with those of transplant patients during the same operation to discharge period. In addition, we were aware of a number of studies which have attempted to cost bypass grafts using different costing methods to those employed here. By presenting our own cost estimates on bypass patients we hope to facilitate any comparison that others may want to make between such studies and our estimates for transplant patients, providing some indication of the extent to which apparent cost differences are substantive or simply attributable to variations in costing methods employed.

We collected prospective information on resource usage and costed 24 patients at Harefield and 47 patients at Papworth in the period January to June 1984. All patients received some form of bypass grafting operation; we have not sought to distinguish between the number or type of grafts received in a given operation.

Both centres display similar periods of inpatient length of stay following bypass grafting, this being 10.3 days for Harefield and 11.1 days at Papworth. TABLE 12.1 presents the cost summary for patients from both centres and it is noticeable that the close similarity in length of stay is reflected in most areas of hospital resource usage. (It should be noted here that postoperative inpatient stay at Harefield does not include any time in the flats; thus enabling more direct comparison between the two centres than the transplant patients.) We estimate the overall operation to discharge cost at Harefield to be £2457 and £1990 at Papworth.

The major difference in costs is the higher nursing cost at Harefield which reflects a longer average period spent in ITU. The difference in operation costs reflects a longer average duration of operation at Harefield.

We would stress that the differences between the centres might well be explained by a different mix of patients. The importance in our context is not the small difference between the two centres, except to the extent that it emphasises that differences in costs between the centres would probably be found for any broad category of patients. Rather the figures provide a rough benchmark of £2.0–£2.5 thousand that can be compared with the costs for transplant patients, of £5.3 at Harefield and £11.2 at Papworth (see TABLE 6.3).

Table 12.1   Average costs per patient of Coronary Artery Bypass Graft Operations. Operation to discharge (1 Jan 1984–30 June 1984)

(1983–84 Prices)

	CABG Operation to Discharge	
	Harefield (N = 24)	Papworth (N = 47)
	£	£
Nursing	628	353
Consumables	63	35
Drugs	87	57
Recipient operation	824	633
Respiratory Physiology	28	—
Radiography etc	64	60
Pathology etc	101	128
Blood Products	185	153
Electrocardiography	19	11
Physiotherapy	16	30
Sub-Total	2014	1461
General Services	443	529
Grand Total	2457	1990

It is not our purpose to review and formally compare our estimates for the costs of CABG with those of others. However despite differences in costing methods our figures for CABG patients at Harefield and Papworth appear to be broadly in line with those estimated in several other studies. Recent British studies which investigated the average cost of CABG, excluding capital, suggest costs in the range of £2500/£4500 in recent years. (Wasfie and Brown [1981]; Wheatley and Dark [1982]; Mollo [1982]). In addition an as yet unpublished review of such costings quotes DHSS estimates of average recurrent cost of CABG (including angiography, but excluding capital) in the range £2546/£3038 at 1983–84 prices. (Williams [1984]). Given that our figures exclude the costs of the time of the surgical team, for consistency with our treatment of heart transplant costs, the estimates tally closely. Indeed they have been costed in rather more detail on rather larger samples than many of the previously quoted figures.

12.3 The benefits to coronary artery bypass graft patients

The Nottingham Health Profile (NHP) was completed by our sample of CABG patients preoperatively and was subsequently administered (usually by post) at three months following the operation. The aim was to provide a "before and after" comparison for such patients, similar to that constructed for transplant patients.

Comparison of responses on Section I of the NHP before, and three months after, bypass grafting are presented in TABLE 12.2 for Harefield and Papworth patients combined using the Wilcoxon test for paired observations. In general the evidence is of significant ($P < 0.01$) improvement in the various dimensions of the NHP with the exception of Energy which indicates no significant improvement ($P = 0.18$).

Health profile responses for transplant and CABG patients were compared both pre-operatively and at three months post-operatively. The results presented in TABLE 12.3 indicate that transplant patients at assessment are significantly ($P < 0.05$) "less healthy" than CABG patients immediately pre-operatively, in four of the six dimensions of Section I of the NHP. No significant difference between the patient groups could be found in the dimensions of Pain ($P = 0.52$) and Emotional Reactions ($P = 0.27$).

The comparisons made between transplant and CABG patients at three months after transplant operation is presented in TABLE 12.4 and results clearly indicate that in no dimension of Section I of the NHP is there evidence of a significant difference in "health" between the two groups of postoperative patients.

Table 12.2   Nottingham Health Profile, Part I: Coronary artery bypass graft patients, paired comparisons (Wilcoxon test) of pre-operative and three-month post-operative patient profiles. Combined hospital data (N = 69)

	Number of ties	Pre-operative mean rank score	Post-operative mean rank score	'Z' statistic	2-tailed P value
Energy	28	22.23	19.26	− 1.34	0.18
Pain	6	33.25	23.38	− 5.62	< 0.01
Emotional reactions	6	33.71	6.75	− 6.72	< 0.01
Sleep	24	26.52	15.21	− 3.44	< 0.01
Social isolation	17	30.48	9.80	− 5.38	< 0.01
Physical mobility	6	33.91	16.71	− 6.10	< 0.01

Table 12.3 **Nottingham Health Profile, Part I: Heart transplants, definitely accepted, at assessment, compared with pre-operative CABG patients (Mann-Whitney U Test)**

	Mean Rank Scores			
	(N = 134) transplant	(N = 80) CABG	Mann-Whitney 'U' statistic	2-tailed P value corrected for ties
Energy	126.51	75.65	2812.0	< 0.01
Pain	105.40	111.02	5078.0	0.52
Emotional reactions	111.09	101.49	4879.0	0.27
Sleep	119.64	87.16	3733.0	< 0.01
Social isolation	114.16	96.34	4467.5	0.04
Physical mobility	119.93	86.68	3694.5	< 0.01

Table 12.4 **Nottingham Health Profile, Part I: Heart transplants, three months posttransplant compared with CABG patients three months postoperation (Mann-Whitney U Test)**

	Mean Rank Scores			
	(N = 71) transplant	(N = 69) CABG	Mann-Whitney 'U' statistic	2-tailed P value corrected for ties
Energy	72.94	67.99	2276.0	0.29
Pain	68.89	72.15	2335.5	0.56
Emotional reactions	67.03	73.01	2207.0	0.30
Sleep	72.69	68.25	2294.0	0.42
Social isolation	65.94	75.19	2126.0	0.08
Physical mobility	69.27	71.77	2362.0	0.69

12.4 Implications for future evaluative research

The difficulty in making comparative judgements about the relative merits of alternative uses of health service resources, is one that concerns us as researchers. From the outset we were concerned to use an existing and validated instrument for the measurement of quality of life, rather than attempt to develop one specifically for this study. We are aware that the Nottingham Health Profile is being incorporated into a growing number of studies. The sample comparison with CABG patients presented here indicates how comparisons can be made.

On the cost side we have endeavoured to use a methodology that is easy to replicate; and have developed an ITU nursing dependency categorisation that can be used alongside Barr's ward nursing categories.

We believe that there is currently a need for a reassessment of whether researchers now have a consistent set of methods and instruments that can be routinely incorporated into future evaluations. It is the commonality of the resulting data collected which will facilitate future comparisons between studies.

12.5 Summary

As benchmarks for comparison with our information on transplant patients, we used the same methods and conventions to cost a group of coronary artery bypass graft patients at each hospital. For the period from operation to discharge the costs were £2.5 thousand at Harefield and £2.0 at Papworth. These compare with the operation to discharge cost for transplant patients of £5.3 and £11.2 at the centres respectively. In all cases the costs exclude those of the surgeons involved.

For the same group of CABG patients, we used the NHP to measure their quality of life. Pre operatively the CABG patients tended to be less "ill" than the transplant patients at assessment particularly in the dimensions of energy, sleep, social isolation and physical mobility. Comparing three month post operative NHP scores for each, there was no significant difference in the "health" of the transplant and CABG patients.

Whilst these figures provide a limited comparative background to help "calibrate" our measures for the heart transplant patients, there is a clear need for more evaluative studies using agreed and consistent methods and conventions to provide full comparative data for other groups of patients.

13.   The Costs and Benefits: An Overview

13.1 Introduction

In the preceding Chapters we have presented a considerable amount of detailed information and analyses on both the costs and benefits of the programmes. We have tried objectively to indicate in detail and methodological strengths and weaknesses. In general however the major weakness is one that is inevitable. All our figures relate to the past—albeit and very recent past. It is a description and analysis of the two programmes up to 1984. Policies need to be concerned with 1985 onwards.

In this final chapter we have tried to bring together some of the main findings and to draw out their implications for the future. In its essence therefore it must be speculative rather than firmly analytical. It should however provide a basis for informed discussion.

13.2 The costs and benefits: A methodological overview

In assessing the strength of our evidence the recurring problem as we have repeatedly stressed is the absence of a formal control group. Without it, sceptics or those requiring indisputable statistical evidence will be able to question the extent to which the benefits and the resource costs result from the procedure. Even some of the comparison groups we initially identified in Chapter One have included very small numbers or have not in practice existed.

We were not able to identify an adequate sub-group of patients who at assessment were found to be medically suitable but excluded on psychosocial or age grounds. The numbers who have received "other" operations during the 30 months of cost data collection were just 13 at Papworth and 4 at Harefield. It was also clear from the details that these patients were not a homogeneous group: for some alternative cardiac surgery was the surgeons' preferred option, for others surgery was a last-ditch procedure performed in the hope that a subsequent heart transplant would thus be made possible.

For comparison therefore, we have had to rely heavily on the postacceptance but pretransplant cost and benefit observations of transplanted patients and of those accepted who died waiting. This approach is very thoroughly discussed particularly in Chapter Eight in the context of the survival analyses.

Arguably the second weakness is that we have not been able to identify a clearly defined cohort of patients and follow them through for several years. We have had to combine cross-sectional and time series analyses to maximise the useful data we could obtain from programmes which, initially at least, involved very small numbers for analysis. As a result our sample sizes inevitably vary. Further variation results from the different considerations that have governed the data collection for different parts of the Report. Where we have any particular reservations about a sample they have been noted. But the strength of this approach is that within a three year study we have been able to build-up a picture that includes the costs and quality of life of the longer-term survivors who were transplanted near the beginning of the programme.

13.3 Benefits

Despite the methodological problems, we believe that the evidence on benefits is very favourable to transplantation. Survival after the operation now appears to have caught up with the results achieved at Stanford. The overall experience since the beginning of the programmes gives survival probabilities of 0.73 for six months, 0.69 for one year, 0.61 for two years, and 0.54 for three years. The short-term survival of patients since 1983 has certainly improved and for those patients the survival probability for six months is 0.82. The problem is in terms of the uncertainty surrounding long-term survival and particularly whether the clear benefits of Cyclosporin A in terms of the longer-term survival pattern will be sustained. The issue of drug side-effects and nephrotoxicity may become important.

The extent to which survival can be further increased is unknown. Detailed covariate analysis may indicate ways of improving survival, perhaps through donor selection. On the other hand, it is not clear to what extent transplantation will prove a long-term solution of IHD patients, or how frequently retransplantation may be needed after a period of time.

The statistical evidence, based on the post-acceptance survival of patients who do not receive a transplant and of the acceptance to transplant survival of those who do, confirms the clinical judgement that on average accepted patients have a prognosis of about nine months without transplant.

In terms of our measures of quality of life there is a very marked and favourable difference between pre and posttransplant scores. This subjective measure of health that we have used, could of course be distorted by feelings of gratitude; *in principle* it could be a dramatic placebo effect. But all the corroborating evidence of the interviews and the clinical studies indicate the reality of the change. There is little reason to expect that this posttransplant quality of life, which is very little restricted and very close to what is normal for the relevant age groups, can be further improved. However again the issue of long-term drug side-effects may effect it.

13.4 Costs

As we have stressed, the cost figures must be a dependent upon the boundaries drawn round them. These tend to be the product of a mixture of institutional organisations, political decisions and historical accident. Such are the dividing lines between the costs that are incurred at, or met by, each of the transplant centres, and costs met by other budgets.

Policy decisions about the future of heart transplantation should reflect a broad definition of costs, certainly including those met by other parts of the NHS. For such purposes, we think that the evidence suggests that the costs of assessment at Harefield (£1200) are a fairer representation of the costs to the NHS as a whole, than those at Papworth, where the surgeons encourage the referring centres to carry out some of the necessary tests.

In the period between assessment and transplant we would argue that there is no evidence of major difference in treatment or tests, from those that would be carried out as part of a normal medical regime for such patients. There may however be a small resource cost in terms of slightly closer monitoring, possibly additional interviews, and perhaps a marginally higher chance of hospitalisation. With a growing knowledge and awareness amongst referring doctors of the selection criteria, and increased selectivity based on referral information, it may be possible to reduce the number of assessments. But to some extent any reductions in formal assessments may be offset by more intensive testing of patients prior to referral. At this stage, again for indicative planning, an assumption of two assessments for every transplant performed seems appropriate.

The *total* costs of the donor operation are very dependent on the assumed cost of associated travel, and the assumptions made as regards those costs that should be more correctly jointly attributed to the procurement of all the organs taken from a particular donor. A planning figure of £1,000 has been adopted here.

For the cost of the period from transplant to discharge including the recipient operation itself, we would argue that the difference in costs between the two centres is significant and not simply a product of arbitrary cost boundaries or the different practice at Papworth of inserting a pacemaker. The detailed figures show that the costing to discharge may exaggerate the cost differences over a longer period, in that the cost of the much higher level of subsequent outpatient visits by Harefield patients begins to erode the cost differential. But even if the costs over the first six months are taken, and allowance made for outpatient visits to other hospitals, the Harefield cost seems still to be significantly lower. For planning purposes we would take the average of the two centres during the most recent "cross section view" including an allowance for outpatient visits elsewhere. This gives a total figure of £12.7 thousand per patient for the first six months. For the next six months the same calculation gives an average figure of £3.1 thousand and for the third six-month period £2.5 thousand. Beyond this point the figures are rather less firm, firstly because of our smaller numbers of patients and secondly because the costs begin to reflect pre-Cyclosporin drug regimes. For planning purposes it may well be appropriate to assume that the full cost to the NHS may well not fall much below £2.5 thousand per six-month period, of which about £1.5 thousand is likely to be the cost of Cyclosporin.

All these figures exclude the costs of the surgical teams, and the social work input. In terms of figures for indicative planning for a future programme not too different in size from the current ones, an annual programme staff cost of £40–45 thousand (excluding research time) would seem to accord with the detailed figures.

13.5 The broad costs of a hypothetical programme

The value of such crude costs is that they can be fitted into a broad-brush cost scheme representing a hypothetical programme.

Let us assume a programme of 60 transplants per year — 60 being merely a convenient figure lying between the current annual rates of transplantation at the two centres — and conceive of it as two cohorts of 30 patients so we can consider costs in six-month periods. The cost of each cohort will depend upon their survival rates, and solely for such an indicative exercise we have taken the combined survival experience of the two centres over four years, adjusted it

Table 13.1 Schematic matrix to estimate the costs of a hypothetical programme of 60 transplants per year based on a crude projecton of survival

Half-year cohorts	Years 1.0		2.0		3.0		4.0		5.0		6.0		7.0		8.0		9.0		10.0		11.0	
Survivors:																						
1	30.0	24.6	23.1	21.6	20.4	19.2	18.0	16.8	15.6	14.4	13.2	12.0	10.8	9.6	8.4	7.2	6.0	4.8	3.6	2.4	1.2	0.0
2		30.0	24.6	23.1	21.6	20.4	19.2	18.0	16.8	15.6	14.4	13.2	12.0	10.8	9.6	8.4	7.2	6.0	4.8	3.6	2.4	1.2
3			30.0	24.6	23.1	21.6	20.4	19.2	18.0	16.8	15.6	14.4	13.2	12.0	10.8	9.6	8.4	7.2	6.0	4.8	3.6	2.4
4				30.0	24.6	23.1	21.6	20.4	19.2	18.0	16.8	15.6	14.4	13.2	12.0	10.8	9.6	8.4	7.2	6.0	4.8	3.6
5					30.0	24.6	23.1	21.6	20.4	19.2	18.0	16.8	15.6	14.4	13.2	12.0	10.8	9.6	8.4	7.2	6.0	4.8
6						30.0	24.6	23.1	21.6	20.4	19.2	18.0	16.8	15.6	14.4	13.2	12.0	10.8	9.6	8.4	7.2	6.0
7							30.0	24.6	23.1	21.6	20.4	19.2	18.0	16.8	15.6	14.4	13.2	12.0	10.8	9.6	8.4	7.2
8								30.0	24.6	23.1	21.6	20.4	19.2	18.0	16.8	15.6	14.4	13.2	12.0	10.8	9.6	8.4
9									30.0	24.6	23.1	21.6	20.4	19.2	18.0	16.8	15.6	14.4	13.2	12.0	10.8	9.6
10										30.0	24.6	23.1	21.6	20.4	19.2	18.0	16.8	15.6	14.4	13.2	12.0	10.8
11											30.0	24.6	23.1	21.6	20.4	19.2	18.0	16.8	15.6	14.4	13.2	12.0
12												30.0	24.6	23.1	21.6	20.4	19.2	18.0	16.8	15.6	14.4	13.2
13													30.0	24.6	23.1	21.6	20.4	19.2	18.0	16.8	15.6	14.4
14														30.0	24.6	23.1	21.6	20.4	19.2	18.0	16.8	15.6
15															30.0	24.6	23.1	21.6	20.4	19.2	18.0	16.8
16																30.0	24.6	23.1	21.6	20.4	19.2	18.0
17																	30.0	24.6	23.1	21.6	20.4	19.2
18																		30.0	24.6	23.1	21.6	20.4
19																			30.0	24.6	23.1	21.6
20																				30.0	24.6	23.1
21																					30.0	24.6
22																						30.0
Number surviving	24.6	47.7	69.3	89.7	108.9	126.9	143.7	159.3	173.7	186.9	198.9	209.7	219.3	227.7	234.9	240.9	245.7	249.3	251.7	252.9	252.9	252.9
Costs: £ Thousand (1983–84) prices																						
New Transplants	381.0	381.0	381.0	381.0	381.0	381.0	381.0	381.0	381.0	381.0	381.0	381.0	381.0	381.0	381.0	381.0	381.0	381.0	381.0	381.0	381.0	381.0
Care of previous cohorts	0.0	76.3	134.0	188.0	239.0	287.0	322.0	374.0	431.0	449.0	482.0	512.0	539.0	563.0	584.0	602.0	617.0	629.0	638.0	644.0	647.0	647.0
Assessments	72.0	72.0	72.0	72.0	72.0	72.0	72.0	72.0	72.0	72.0	72.0	72.0	72.0	72.0	72.0	72.0	72.0	72.0	72.0	72.0	72.0	72.0
Donor operations	30.0	30.0	30.0	30.0	30.0	30.0	30.0	30.0	30.0	30.0	30.0	30.0	30.0	30.0	30.0	30.0	30.0	30.0	30.0	30.0	30.0	30.0
Programme staff	22.5	22.5	22.5	22.5	22.5	22.5	22.5	22.5	22.5	22.5	22.5	22.5	22.5	22.5	22.5	22.5	22.5	22.5	22.5	22.5	22.5	22.5
Half-year total	505.5	581.8	639.5	693.5	744.5	792.5	837.5	879.5	918.5	954.5	987.5	1017.5	1044.5	1068.5	1089.5	1107.5	1122.5	1134.5	1143.5	1149.5	1152.5	1152.5
Annual cost	1087.3		1333.0		1537.0		1717.0		1873.0		2005.0		2113.0		2197.0		2257.0		2293.0		2305.0	

156

upwards to reflect the higher (short-term) survival that has been achieved since 1983 and then crudely extrapolated the survival in a linear fashion. This gives a rather ungenerous theoretical maximum survival of 11 years; this assumption as applied to a cohort of 30 transplant patients is shown as the first row in TABLE 13.1. With a steady "flow" of cohorts of 30 new transplants every six months, and with an unchanging survival curve, the "stock" of surviving patients steadily increases until a "steady-state" is reached after 11 years with approximately 250 patients surviving. With more favourable initial survival assumptions, or with improving survival probabilities, the number would increase and the steady-state would be delayed.

If the flow of new patients and the stock of existing patients is costed using the crude averages we indicated then the annual cost in constant 1983–1984 prices will rise from approximately £1.1 million in the first year to £2.3 million in the eleventh and subsequent years. What we wish to stress at this point is the general nature of this build-up effect rather than the specific, and inevitably arguable, figures.

This growing real cost of a programme with a constant annual number of transplants needs to be appreciated. In resource terms the workload of routine posttransplant check-ups needs to be carefully and explicitly planned for. The increase in cost is, of course, only the mirror image of the increasing number of high quality life-years being saved. The annual benefits too would be increasing over the ten years until the "steady state" is reached.

From our cost information it is very difficult to draw out any firm implications for the most cost-effective scale for a programme. However a number of observations should be made. Firstly in terms of buildings and capital that are needed, the requirements are little differentiated from those for other major cardiac surgery. This suggests that to try to separate the transplantation programmes from the other cardiac work in a centre may simply reduce the efficiency with which the whole stock of capital and equipment can be used. On the other hand the undoubted skills and experience of the current transplant teams and all the associated staff in the hospitals needs to be used to the full. The two programmes have improved both their effectiveness (in terms of patient survival etc) and the cost-effectiveness of their use of resources. A new centre elsewhere would almost certainly have to start further back on the "learning curve".

13.6 Costing and funding

These rather crude programme cost figures are merely indicative, and should be used only to explore the longer-term costs of a hypothetical programme to the NHS as a whole. They are clearly inappropriate to detailed financial allocation to, or within the transplant centres. Even our detailed costings need to be treated very cautiously in terms of allocation of funds to different departments. For such a purpose, a detailed and specific consideration is needed of where the costs will fall, and their impact at the margin.

For such funding to be realistic, it needs to relate to an agreed policy as to which costs of the programme should be met within the centres and which are going to be allowed, or encouraged, to fall elsewhere. For example our costs include all drug costs although post-discharge they will not normally be dispensed from the hospital.

157

In the planning model, costs at the donor hospital are included. If specific funding is provided, its level must reflect these factors in accordance with the detailed local arrangements. To the extent that any agreed arrangements differ between the centres then the funding should also do so.

The long term check-ups and follow-up of the increasing number of survivors, in particular will need to be allowed for in any funding, on the basis of an agreed policy as to where, and by whom, this follow-up will be carried out. Close collaboration with other regional cardiac centres might be an efficient way to do this.

13.7 Monitoring and change

Over the three years of our study there has been considerable change. Costs, particularly at Harefield, have fallen, and survival at both centres has steadily improved. Selection criteria have been amended to reflect new knowledge; heart-lung transplantation has started (although no data on these is included in this *Report*). A number of other possible changes and developments may be just over the horizon. The artificial heart as a temporary holding device prior to transplantation, or as a totally implantable alternative to a donor organ may not be far away. We cannot hope to predict these changes, but we can be confident that change will occur.

What we have observed in terms of costs and in terms of quantitative and qualitative benefits will similarly continue to change. Whilst a research study of the sort that we have undertaken cannot be continued indefinitely, it would seem essential that a formal, though possibly internal, monitoring of the two programmes (and any others, if there be such) should be an integral part of the programmes. It would contribute to our knowledge of the procedure and its benefits, encourage cost-effectiveness, and monitor changes in the costs relative to the benefits, as perhaps techniques change, new immunosuppressive drugs become available, or patient selection criteria are altered or relaxed (for instance, if further paediatric work is done at Harefield). Such changes need to be monitored and assessed.

We have noted a healthy competitiveness between the two centres, perhaps aided or abetted by our joint study. Certainly we believe that we have made the centres even more cost conscious and our data have probably influenced behaviour. There is no reason to suppose that future financial arrangements will require anything other than continuing attention to costs. But we would hope that comparative information continues to be produced, albeit in rather less detail. It would be vital information from any new centre be included.

13.8 The final judgement

This Report can only help in making a decision as to whether more or less should in future be spent on the programmes. We are left with little doubt of the effectiveness of the procedure in terms of the improvement in quality and quantity of life of transplanted patients. But the value of these benefits must be compared with the value of the potential benefits to other, perhaps quite different, patients elsewhere — benefits that will have to be foregone in using resources from a given total NHS budget for heart transplantation rather than some other purpose. The comparisons are a matter of judgement. Certainly they should not be arbitrary, and it is to be hoped that they will not be a matter of mere political expediency. Nor should they be emotionally overlaid with the drama of transplantation. It was suggested to us in one centre that the procedure should now be seen as "a routine cardiac operation that happens to be a transplant". The benefits and costs we have observed, or projected forwards, need to be set against comparable evidence for other procedures or services competing for funds. For some such services there is well documented, if not methodologically identical, information on costs and benefits. For others there is firm evidence at least of effectiveness in terms of some positive patient benefit. However, some services remain essentially unevaluated. The evidence of this *Report* should help to make the comparison with other well evaluated services easier. It is not for us to prejudge in whose favour the comparison will be. But hopefully, it will help to prevent demands for resources from services of unassessed benefit and unmeasured cost depriving the transplant programmes of resources that they can clearly use to benefit their patients.

References

AITKIN M; LAIRD N, and FRANCIS B [1983] 'A Reanalysis of the Stanford Heart Transplant Data' *Journal of the American Statistical Association,* vol 78, no 382, pp 264–274

AYDELOTTE M K [1973]
Nursing Staffing Methodology — A Review and Critique of Selected Literature DHEW Publication, no (NIH) 73.433, US Department of Health Education and Welfare, Washington DC

BACKET E M; McEWEN J, and HUNT S M [1981]
Health and Quality of Life: End of Grant Report to SSRC (HR 6157/1) (mimeo)

BARR A [1964]
'Measuring Nursing Care' in McLachlan G (ed) *Problems and Progress in Medical Care,* Nuffield Provincial Hospitals Trust

BARR A; MOORES B, and RHYS-HEARN C [1973]
'A Review of the Various Methods of Measuring the Dependency of Patients on Nursing Staff' *International Journal of Nursing Studies,* vol 10, pp 195–208

BAUMANN B [1961]
'Diversities in Conceptions of Health and Physical Fitness' *Journal of Health and Human Behaviour,* vol 2, no 1, pp 39–46

BERGNER M, *et al* [1976a]
'The Sickness Impact Profile: Conceptual Formulation and Methodology for the Development of a Health Status Measure' *International Journal of Health Services,* vol 6, no 3, pp 393–415

BERGNER M, *et al* [1978b]
'The Sickness Impact Profile: Validation of a Health Status Measure' *Medical Care,* vol XIV, no 1, pp 57–67

BRESLOW N [1970]
'A generalized Kruskal-Wallis test for comparing k samples subject to unequal patterns of censorship' *Biometrika,* vol 57, pp 579–594

BRITISH CARDIAC SOCIETY [1984]
'Report on Cardiac Transplantation in the United Kingdom', *British Heart Journal,* vol 52, pp 679–682

BRITISH HEART FOUNDATION [1980]
Can we Justify the Costs of Cardiac Surgery and Pacemaking? Proceedings of the British Heart Foundation Symposium, Newcastle-upon-Tyne, 19 June 1980 Tillots Laboratories, Bedfordshire, England

BUCKLEY J, and JAMES I [1979]
'Linear Regression with censored Data' *Biometrika,* vol 66, pp 429–436

BUSH J W; BLISCHKE W R, and BERRY C C [1975]
'Health Indices, Outcomes and the Quality of Medical Care' in Yaffe R and Zalkind D (eds) *Evaluation in Health Services Delivery,* New York, Engineering Foundation, pp 313–339

BUXTON M J [1983]
'The economics of heart transplantation programmes: measuring the benefits' in Teeling-Smith [1983]

CLARK D A , *et la* [1971]
'Prognosis of Patients Selected for Cardiac Transplantation' *Annals of Internal Medicine,* vol 75, no 1, pp 15–21

COX D R [1972]
'Regression Models and Life-tables' *Journal of the Royal Statistical Society — Series B,* vol 34, no 2, pp 187–202

COX D R and OAKES D [1984]
Analysis of Survival Data Chapman and Hall

CROWLEY J, and HU M [1974]
'Covariance Analysis of Heart Transplant Survival Data' *Journal of American Statistical Association,* vol 77, no 357, pp 27–36

CULYER A; LAVERS A, and WILLIAMS A [1971]
'Social Indicators: Health' *Social Trends,* vol 2, pp 31–42

CULYER A (ed) [1983]
Health Indicators Martin Robertson and Company Ltd.

CUTLER S J and EDERER F [1958]
'Maximum Utilisation of the Life-table method in Analysing Survival' *Journal of Chronic diseases,* vol 8, pp 699–713

DIXON W J [1983]
BMDP Statistical Software: 1983 Revised Printing University of California Press

DHSS [1979]
Health Services Management: Charges for Private Residents and Non-Resident Patients HN(79)28, DHSS, London

DHSS [1981]
Whole Hospital Costs Cost Intelligence Service Note, 6061, June, DHSS, London

DHSS [1984a]
Handling charges for Blood and Blood Derivatives Supplied to Non-NHS Hospitals, HC(84)5, March, DHSS, London

DHSS [1984b]
Hospital cost Returns for the Year Ending March 1983, HMSO, 1984

ENGLISH T A H [1978]
'United Kingdom Cardiac surgical Register: Report on a Pilot Study,' *Thorax,* vol 33, pp 131–132

ENGLISH T A H [1982]
'Cardiac Transplantation' *Hospital Update,* vol 8, no 11, pp 1447–1454

ENGLISH T A H; COOPER D K, and CORY-PEARCE R [1980]
'Recent Experience with Heart Transplantation' *British Medical Journal,* vol 281, 13 September, pp 699–702

ENGLISH T A H; CORY-PEARCE R, and McGREGOR C [1982]
'Heart Transplantation at Papworth Hospital' *Heart Transplantation,* vol 1, no 2, pp 110–111

ENGLISH T A H, *et al* [1984a]
'Selection and procurement of Hearts for Transplantation' *British Medical Journal,* vol 288, 23 June, pp 1889–1891

ENGLISH T A H, *et al* [1984b]
'The UK Cardiac Surgical Register, 1977–1982', *British Medical Journal,* vol 289, 3 November, pp 1205–1208

EVANS R W [1982a]
'Economic and Social Costs of Heart Transplantation' *Heart Transplantation,* vol 1, no 3, pp 243–251

EVANS R W [1982b]
Dimensions of Family Impact Pertinent to Heart Transplantation National Heart Transplantation Study: Update no 8, June 22 (mimeo)

FABRAY C E [1983]
Methods of Measuring Work and Costing Activity in Pathology Departments, Financial Information Project Working Paper No 83/01, WMRHA, Birmingham

GAIL M H [1972]
'Does Cardiac Transplantation Prolong Life? *Annals of Internal Medicine,* vol 76, no 5, pp 815–817

GOODWIN J F [1984]
Personal Communication

HARBERMAN S [1980]
'Puting a Price on Life' *Health and Social Services Journal,* July 4, pp 877–879

HARPER D R [1975]
Comparative Disease Costing in Surgical Patients MD Thesis, University of Aberdeen

HARRIS A I [1971]
Handicapped and Impaired in Great Britain Part I Office of Population, Censuses and Surveys: Social Survey Division, HMSO, London

HELLINGER F [1982]
'An Analysis of a Public Program for Heart Transplantation' *Journal of Human Resources,* vol XVII, no 2, pp 307–313

HUNT S M; McKENNA S P, and McEWEN J [1981]
The Nottingham Health Profile: Manual, (mimeo)

HUNT S M, *et al* [1982]
'Subjective Health of Patients with Peripheral Vascular Disease' *The Practitioner,* vol 226, January, pp 133–136

HUNT S M, *et al* [forthcoming]
'Subjective Health Assessments and the Perceived Outcome of Minor Surgery' *Journal of Psychosomatic Research*

JAMIESON S E, *et al* [1979]
'Current Management of Cardiac Transplant Recipients' *British Heart Journal,* vol 42, pp 703–708

KALBFLEISCH J, and PRENTICE R L [1980]
The Statistical Analysis of Failure Time Data Wiley, New York

KAPLAN E L, and MEIER P [1980]
'Nonparametric Estimation from Incomplete Observations' *Journal of American Statistical Association,* vol 53, pp 475–481
KAPLAN R M; BUSH J W and BERRY C C [1976]
'Health Status: Types of Validity and Index of Well-being' *Health Services Research,* Winter, pp 478–507
KIND P [1982]
'A comparison of two models for scaling health indicators' *International Journal of Epidemiology,* vol 11, no 3, 1982, pp 271–275
KOUL H; SUSARTA V, and VAN RYZIN J [1981]
'Regression Analysis with Randomly Right Censored Data' *Annals of Statistics,* vol 9, pp 1276–1288
MANTEL N [1966]
'Evaluation of Survival Data and Two New Rank Order Statistics Arising in its consideration' *Cancer Chemotherapy Reports,* vol 50, no 3, pp 163–170
MARTINI C J, and McDOWELL I [1976]
'Health Status: Patient and Physician Judgements' *Health Services Research,* vol 11, Winter, pp 508–515
McDOWELL I W; MARTINI C J M, and WAUGH W [1978]
'A Method for Self-assessment of Disability Before and After Hip-replacement Operations' *British Medical Journal,* 23 September, pp 857–859
McEWEN J [1983]
'The Nottingham Health Profile: a measure of perceived health' in *Measuring the Social Benefits of Medicine,* Teeling-Smith (ed) Office of Health Economics, pp 75–84
McKENNA S P; HUNT S M, and McEWEN J [1981]
'Weighting the Seriousness of Perceived Health Problems using Thurstone's method of Paired Comparisons' *International Journal of Epidemiology,* vol 10, no 1, pp 93–97
MESSMER B J, *et al* [1969]
'Survival Times after Cardiac Allografts' *Lancet,* no 1, pp 954–956
MILLER R G [1976]
'Least Squares Regression with Censored Data' *Biometrika* vol 63, pp 449–464
MILLER R G, and HALPERN J [1982]
'Regression with censored Data' *Biometrika,* vol 69, no 3, pp 521–531
MINISTRY OF HEALTH [1963]
Pathology Measurement of Work in Units, Hospital O and M Service Reports, HMSO London
MITCHELL M; GODDEN E, and BALK T [1977]
'The Aberdeen Formula: a Trial in S E Thames' *Nursing Times Occasional Papers,* vol 73, pp 839–840
MOLLO S [1982]
'Toward Better Costing' *Health and Social Service Journal,* March 18, pp 339–341
MOSER C A; KALTON G [1971]
Survey Methods in Social Investigation Second Edition, London: Heinemann
NAJMAN J M, and LEVINE S [1981]
'Evaluating the Impact of Medical Care and Technologies on the Quality of Life: A Review and Critique' *Social Science and Medicine,* vol 15F, pp 107–115

NORTH EAST METROPOLITAN REGIONAL HOSPITAL BOARD
(NEMRHB) [1972]
*Draft Report on the Evaluation of the Intensive Therapy Unit of Whipps Cross
Hospital* Draft Report 341, Management Services Division NEMRHB, London
NORWICH H S, and SENIOR O E [1971]
'Determining Nursing Establishment' *Nursing Times Occasional Papers,* vol 67,
pp 17–20
Office of Population Censuses and Surveys [1984]
Hospital Inpatient Enquiry: 1982 Summary Tables, HMSO, London
PATRICK D [1980]
'Standardization of Comparative Health Status Measures: Using Scales de-
veloped in America in an English Speaking Country' in *Proceedings of the Third
Biennial Conference on Health Survey Research Methods,* (Reston, Va; 17th
May 1980), published by National Centre for Health Services Research, US
DHSS, Publication no PHS 81–3268, pp 216–220
PATRICK D (ed) [1981]
The Longitudinal Disability Interview Survey: Phase I Report Social Medicine
and Health Services Research Unit, St. Thomas's Hospital Medical School,
London
PATRICK D (ed) [1982]
The Longitudinal Disability Interview Survey: Phase II Report Social Medicine
and Health Services Research Unit, St. Thomas's Hospital Medical School,
London
PENNOCK J L, *et al* [1982]
'Cardiac Transplantation in Perspective for the Future: Survival, Compli-
cations, Rehabilitation, and Cost' *Journal of Thoracic and Cardiovascular
Surgery,* vol 83, pp 168–177
RAY C; LINDOP J, and GIBSON S [1982]
'The Concept of Coping' *Psychological Medicine,* vol 12, pp 385–395
REITZ B A, and STINSON E B [1982]
'Cardiac Transplantation — 1982' *Journal of the American Medical Associ-
ation,* vol 248, no 10, pp 1225–1227
RHYS-HEARN C [1974]
'Evaluation of Patients' Nursing Needs: Prediction of Staffing' *Nursing Times
Occasional Papers,* vol 70, pp 69–84
RHYS-HEARN C [1979]
'Comparison of the Rhys-Hearn Method of Determining Nursing Staff Require-
ments with the Aberdeen Formula' *International Journal of Nursing Studies,*
vol 16, pp 95–103
ROSS J K, *et al* [1978]
'Wessex Cardiac Surgery Follow-up Survey: the Quality of Life After Oper-
ation' *Thorax,* vol 33, p 3–9
ROSS J K, *et al* [1981]
'The Quality of Life After Cardiac Surgery' *British Medical Journal,* 7 Feb-
ruary, pp 451–453
RUSSELL E M [1974]
Patient Costing Study Scottish Health Sevice Studies, no 31, SHHD, Edinburgh

SACKETT D L, *et al* [1977]
'The Development and Application of Indices of Health: General Methods and a Summary of Results' *American Journal of Public Health,* vol 67, pp 423–428
SCOTTISH HOME AND HEALTH DEPARTMENT [1969]
Nursing Workload Per Patient as a Basis for Staffing Scottish Health services Studies, no 9, SHHD, Edinburgh
SCOTTISH HOME AND HEALTH DEPARTMENT [1984]
Scottish Health statistics: 1982, HMSO
SIEGEL S [1956]
Nonparametric Statistics for the Behavioural Sciences International Student Edition, McGraw Hill, Kogakusha Ltd
SIMMONS R G; KLEIN S K; SIMMONS R L [1977]
Gift of Life: The Social and Psychological Impact of Organ Transplantation New York: Wiley Inter Science
STILWELL, J A [1981]
'Costs of a Clinical Chemistry Laboratory', *Clinical Pathology,* vol 34, pp 589–594
TEELING-SMITH, G (ed) [1983]
Measuring the Social Benefits of Medicines Office of Health Economics, London
THURSTONE L L [1927]
'A Law of Comparative Judgement' *Psychological Review,* vol 34, pp 273–286
TORGERSON W S [1958]
Theory and Methods of Scaling New York: John Wiley
TURNBULL B W; BROWN B W, and HU M [1974]
'Survivorship analysis of Heart Transplant Data' *Journal of American Statistical Association,* vol 69, no 345, pp 74–80
UK TRANSPLANT SERVICE [1982]
Annual Review 1982, UKTS, Bristol
WASFIE T J, and BROWN A H [1981]
The Practitioner, vol 225, pp 739–744
WHEATLEY D J, and DARK J H [1982]
The Practitioner, vol 226, pp 435–440
WHITT C N [1982]
Notes on Work Measurement: Radiology services, Financial Information Project Working Paper No 82/03, WMRHA, Birmingham
WILLIAMS A [1981]
'Welfare Economics and Health Status Measurement' in van der Gaag J and Perlman M (eds) *Health, Economics, and Health Economics,* Amsterdam, North Holland
WILLIAMS A [1984]
Coronary Artery Bypass Grafts: Economic Appraisal, Paper presented to the Consensus Development Conference on CABG, London, Mimeo
WILLIAMS R G A [1979]
'Theories and Measurement in Disability' *Journal of Epidemiology and Community Medicine,* vol 33, pp 32–44
WILLIAMS R G A , *et al* [1976]
'Disability: a Model and Measurement Technique' *British Journal of Preventive and Social Medicine,* vol 30, p 71–78

WRIGHT K G; CAIRNS J A, and SNELL M C [1981]
Costing Care University of Sheffield Joint Unit for Social Services Research
Monograph: Research in Practice, Sheffield

STUDY OF THE COSTS AND BENEFITS
OF THE CARDIAC TRANSPLANTATION PROGRAMMES AT
PAPWORTH AND HAREFIELD HOSPITALS

HEALTH PROFILE

NAME:
DATE OF COMPLETION:
PLEASE RETURN TO:　　　　Mr. S. Gibson,
　　　　　　　　　　　　Research Officer,
　　　　　　　　　　　　DHSS Research Project,
　　　　　　　　　　　　Harefield Hospital,
　　　　　　　　　　　　Harefield,
　　　　　　　　　　　　Middlesex.

This study is supported by DHSS research grants to Brunel University and the University of Cambridge.

LISTED BELOW ARE SOME PROBLEMS PEOPLE MAY HAVE IN THEIR DAILY LIFE.
LOOK DOWN THE LIST AND PUT A TICK IN THE BOX ☑ UNDER <u>YES</u> FOR ANY PROBLEM YOU HAVE AT THE MOMENT.
TICK THE BOX UNDER <u>NO</u> FOR ANY PROBLEM YOU DO NOT HAVE.

<u>PLEASE ANSWER EVERY QUESTION.</u> IF YOU ARE NOT SURE WHETHER TO SAY YES OR NO, TICK WHICHEVER ANSWER YOU THINK IS <u>MORE TRUE</u> AT THE MOMENT.

	YES	NO
I'm tired all the time	☐	☐
I have pain at night	☐	☐
Things are getting me down	☐	☐

	YES	NO
I have unbearable pain	☐	☐
I take tablets to help me sleep	☐	☐
I've forgotten what it's like to enjoy myself	☐	☐

	YES	NO
I'm feeling on edge	☐	☐
I find it painful to change position	☐	☐
I feel lonely	☐	☐

	YES	NO
I can only walk about indoors	☐	☐
I find it hard to bend	☐	☐
Everything is an effort	☐	☐

Please turn over

168

	YES	NO
I'm waking up in the early hours of the morning	☐	☐
I'm unable to walk at all	☐	☐
I'm finding it hard to make contact with people	☐	☐

	YES	NO
The days seem to drag	☐	☐
I have trouble getting up and down stairs or steps	☐	☐
I find it hard to reach for things	☐	☐

REMEMBER IF YOU ARE NOT SURE WHETHER TO ANSWER YES OR NO TO A PROBLEM, TICK WHICHEVER ANSWER YOU THINK IS <u>MORE TRUE</u> AT THE MOMENT.

	YES	NO
I'm in pain when I walk	☐	☐
I lose my temper easily these days	☐	☐
I feel there is nobody I am close to	☐	☐

	YES	NO
I lie awake for most of the night	☐	☐
I feel as if I'm losing control	☐	☐
I'm in pain when I'm standing	☐	☐

Please turn over

PLEASE DO NOT WRITE IN THIS MARGIN

	YES	NO
I find it hard to dress myself	☐	☐
I soon run out of energy	☐	☐
I find it hard to stand for long (e.g. at the kitchen sink, waiting for a bus)	☐	☐

	YES	NO
I'm in constant pain	☐	☐
It takes me a long time to get to sleep	☐	☐
I feel I am a burden to people	☐	☐

	YES	NO
Worry is keeping me awake at night	☐	☐
I feel that life is not worth living	☐	☐
I sleep badly at night	☐	☐

	YES	NO
I'm finding it hard to get on with people	☐	☐
I need help to walk about outside (e.g. a walking aid or someone to support me)	☐	☐
I'm in pain when going up and down stairs or steps	☐	☐

	YES	NO
I wake up feeling depressed	☐	☐
I'm in pain when I'm sitting	☐	☐

NOW WE WOULD LIKE YOU TO THINK ABOUT THE ACTIVITIES IN YOUR LIFE WHICH MAY BE AFFECTED BY HEALTH PROBLEMS. PLEASE TURN OVER AND ANSWER THE NEXT SECTION OF THE QUESTIONNAIRE.

IN THE LIST BELOW, TICK YES FOR EACH ACTIVITY IN YOUR
LIFE WHICH IS BEING AFFECTED BY YOUR STATE OF HEALTH.
TICK NO FOR EACH ACTIVITY WHICH IS NOT BEING AFFECTED.
OR WHICH DOES NOT APPLY TO YOU.

IS YOUR PRESENT STATE OF HEALTH CAUSING PROBLEMS
WITH YOUR...

                                                    YES   NO

JOB OF WORK
(That is, paid employment)   ☐   ☐

LOOKING AFTER THE HOME
Examples: cleaning and cooking, repairs,   ☐   ☐
odd jobs around the home etc.)

SOCIAL LIFE
(Examples: going out, seeing friends,   ☐   ☐
going to the pub etc.)

HOME LIFE
(That is: relationships with   ☐   ☐
other people in your home)

SEX LIFE   ☐   ☐

INTERESTS & HOBBIES
(Examples: sports, arts and crafts,   ☐   ☐
do-it-yourself etc.)

HOLIDAYS
(Examples: summer or winter   ☐   ☐
holidays, weekends away etc.)

NOW PLEASE GO BACK TO PAGE 1 AND
MAKE SURE YOU HAVE ANSWERED YES
OR NO TO EVERY QUESTION ON ALL FOUR PAGES.

Printed in the UK for HMSO, Dd.738705, C9, 4/85.